Ethics and Economics
of Assisted Reproduction

The Cost of Longing

MAURA A. RYAN

GEORGETOWN UNIVERSITY PRESS / WASHINGTON, D.C.

Georgetown University Press, Washington, D.C.
© 2001 by Georgetown University Press. All rights reserved.
Printed in the United States of America

10   9   8   7   6   5   4   3   2   1   2001

This volume is printed on acid-free offset book paper.

Chapter 3 is reprinted with permission of the Society of
Christian Ethics. The original publication is Maura A. Ryan,
"Particular Sorrows, Common Challenges: Infertility and the
Common Good," *The Annual, Society of Christian Ethics*
(1994): 187–206.

Chapter 4 is reprinted with permission from the *Valparaiso
University Law Review.* The original publication is Maura A.
Ryan, "Cloning, Generic Engineering, and the Limits of Procreative Liberty," *Valparaiso University Law Review* 32, no. 2
(1998): 753–71.

For Paul,
and for my family

*Blessed is she who believed that the promise made her
By the Lord would be fulfilled.*
—Luke 1:45

Library of Congress Cataloging-in-Publication Data

Ryan, Maura A., 1957-
    Ethics and economics of assisted reproduction : the cost of longing / Maura A.
Ryan.
        p. cm.—(Moral traditions and moral arguments series)
    Includes index.
    ISBN 0-87840-871-1 (cloth : alk. paper)
    1. Human reproductive technology—Moral and ethical aspects. 2. Human repro-
ductive technology—Economic aspects. 3. Infertitity—Moral and ethical aspects.
4. Infertility—Economic aspects. I. Title. II. Moral traditions & moral arguments.

RG133.5 .R926 2001
176—dc21   2001023258

Contents

Preface

I began thinking about assisted reproduction when I was in graduate school. The ethical questions raised by what were then called the "new" reproductive technologies joined, in fascinating and complicated ways, my interests in feminism, medical ethics, and Roman Catholic moral theology. I became especially intrigued by the questions of distributive justice posed by the expensive pursuit of parenthood in the United States, where we do not guarantee universal access to health care. In trying to ask whether a just society is obliged to help people overcome infertility, I found no shortage of passionate positions but little in the way of satisfying argument.

When I first took up the questions that I explore in this book, infertility was an abstract theoretical problem for me, a device for thinking about how feminist commitments to empowering women and Catholic commitments to the common good intersect in defining the character of procreative liberty and procreative agency. By the time this book went to press, I was the exhausted but awed mother of five-month-old twins from, as someone I know put it, "the Clomid side of the family."[1] In between, I got married, set out to have children, and discovered to my great surprise that I was infertile. No longer just a phenomenon to be studied, infertility became a daily companion and infertility treatment a journey I embarked upon reluctantly but also, in a way, passionately.

Some readers will be disappointed that I did not come away from my professional and personal encounters with assisted reproduction convinced of the unequivocal danger of reproductive technologies for women. To be sure, I have always found the feminist critique of reproductive technologies compelling and continue to view the fertility industry with a healthy skepticism. I am especially troubled by the potentially dangerous symbiosis between the economic interests of fertility specialists in this multimillion dollar business and the often obsessive drive for a child underlying choices about treatment.

Moreover, my experience as a patient has caused me to be more acutely aware, rather than less, of the serious and continually evolving moral questions raised by these technologies.

And yet, reflecting on that experience and the experience of infertile couples I have known, I can only conclude that reproductive technologies are a genuinely mixed blessing. I was grateful to be diagnosed as infertile at a time when there were choices. I understand well why so many infertile couples are willing to count the considerable sacrifices of time, money, control, and intimacy involved in infertility treatment worth it in the end. One does not need to give birth to experience the pure, transformative joy that comes with parenthood or to discover inside that unexpected capacity for love your children call forth. Still, I will always be grateful that I had the privilege of feeling my daughters coming fully into being within me and the chance to pass on the gift of life.

But I also now know intimately something I only glimpsed before, that no one goes through assisted reproduction unscarred. Feminists have written of the "construction of desperation," the crushing social pressures on women to take on the maternal role and the vulnerability of infertile women in the face of them. Others have written of the frightening internal momentum of infertility treatment, where one alternative simply follows the next as though there is no real decision to be made except to stay in the game. Individuals can be more or less at the mercy of those forces, but they are real. I was continually surprised at how little protection education and carefully cultivated professional objectivity afforded when the waves of longing and self-doubt threatened to overtake me.

Reflection on experience has an important place in feminist theory. In urging women to find their own voices, to trust their own instincts, feminism has been concerned, among other things, with unmasking the false objectivity that has characterized much academic literature. The view is always from somewhere, we are reminded, and underneath the generic "man" and "woman" are individual men and women, defined and differentiated by realities such as race, class, sexual orientation, geography, and religion, and by the particular relationships and events that shape their perception and imagination. If I had written this book before my journey through infertility, it would have been a different book. I might have drawn the same conclusions, but it would have been a different book nonetheless. It has been important, therefore, to allow the experience of infertility, my own as well as that of other infertile women, to speak, not as a limit to what questions could be asked, but rather as a kind of touchstone, a locus for testing the assumptions brought to bear and the claims made. If a useful distance is thereby lost, it seems a fair bargain.

Many people helped me in writing this book. Margaret Farley directed my dissertation and has continued to provide support and advice in this and many other projects. Jim Keenan, Paul Lauritzen, Cristy Traina, and Cynthia

Cohen were good enough to read the entire manuscript. Not all of their suggestions were incorporated, but all were appreciated. Gene Outka, Richard Fern, John Paris, Lainie Ross, Ann Dudley Goldblatt, Blake Leyerle, Hindy Najman, and Diane Ryan have all been valuable conversation partners at points along the way. My colleagues and students at the College of the Holy Cross and the University of Notre Dame have often reminded me why I took up this calling. The late Richard McCormick, S.J., was a generous and challenging mentor, and his influence is manifest throughout this project. A visiting faculty fellowship at the MacLean Center for Clinical Medical Ethics at the University of Chicago and a research fellowship at the Center for Research on Women and Gender, University of Illinois-Chicago, gave me supportive and interesting contexts in which to discuss questions of justice in assisted reproduction. Alan LaRue and Shirley Bach invited me to talk through some of my ideas with a wonderful group of people at the Center for the Study of Ethics in Society at Western Michigan University. John Samples and Gail Grella of Georgetown University Press encouraged me to publish this project. David Weiss, Maria Malkiewicz, and James Ball provided research assistance. Zvi Binor, M.D., and the staff at Women's Health Consultants showed me a model of compassionate and self-reflective care. My family encouraged me and even offered to read the book when it was done if I promised to keep it short. My daughters Annie and Meggie graciously postponed reaching any real milestones while I was trying to finish, and my husband Paul Weithman lent love and support of every kind.

NOTE

1 Clomid (clomiphine citrate) is a fertility drug that carries a possible side effect of an increased chance for multiple birth. Most multiple births associated with Clomid are twins.

The danger is not lest the soul should doubt
whether there is any bread, but lest, by a lie,
it should persuade itself that it is not hungry.
It can only persuade itself of this by lying,
for the reality of its hunger is not a belief,
it is a certainty.

—Simone Weil, *Waiting for God*

Introduction

Couples who consulted an infertility expert in depression-era America found themselves facing a time-consuming and often expensive course of diagnosis and treatment. . . . The price of infertility treatment, both financial and otherwise, could be quite steep. A single office visit to a specialist could cost fifteen dollars, and hormonal therapy in the days before the availability of synthetic preparations could run into hundreds of dollars. [Patients were sometimes required] to devote an entire week to the initial diagnostic workup, going from office to office, making love at precisely prescribed intervals, and having their bodily fluids—blood, urine, semen—tested and retested. [Often they came from outside the urban areas where specialists could be found] so to the expense of the physicians' bills and laboratory tests [were] added hotel charges and perhaps lost wages.

—Margaret Marsh and Wanda Ronner, *The Empty Cradle*

In many ways, there has been a revolution in the treatment of infertility since the 1930s. The introduction of in vitro fertilization (IVF) twenty years ago dramatically expanded clinical options, offering new possibilities for overcoming some of the most vexing reproductive problems such as severe endometriosis, premature ovarian failure, and "unexplained infertility." More recently, the development of intracytoplasmic sperm injection (ICSI) has brought genuine breakthroughs in the treatment of male factor infertility, where for many patients traditional medical and surgical treatments were little better than boxer shorts and cold showers. With the advent of gestational surrogacy, even women who have undergone hysterectomies now have the possibility of genetically related children. New techniques for freezing oocytes and the growth

1

of egg donation programs promise to turn back or even *turn off* the biological clock, allowing women to give birth well past natural menopause.

Yet, Margaret Marsh and Wanda Ronner's description could easily apply to couples seeking treatment for infertility in the United States today. A half-century later, infertility treatment remains costly, time-consuming, invasive, and emotionally and physically arduous. Although free-standing clinics are on the rise, specialists are still concentrated in large urban areas. Diagnosis and treatment often involve many appointments over the course of several years, and those at a distance still pay dearly in miles traveled and hours lost. Whether undergoing relatively low-tech therapies such as intrauterine insemination or highly sophisticated procedures such as in vitro fertilization, today's typical infertility patient receives drug therapy to increase the number of eggs produced, in the course of which she assumes the burden of self-administered injections and the risks of ovarian hyperstimulation and multiple gestation. For all the effort, slightly more than half who enter treatment will succeed, if success is measured by a live birth.[1]

From 1988 to 1995, there was a 25 percent increase in the incidence of reported infertility in U.S. women of childbearing age, from 4.9 million to 6.1 million.[2] In the same period of time, infertility-related office visits nearly tripled and expenditures for in vitro fertilization alone in the United States grew from 66 million in 1987 to more than 200 million in 1997.[3] Most of the costs are borne by patients themselves, some of whom will go heavily into debt, exhaust their savings, or dip into retirement accounts to finance their treatment. Insurance coverage of infertility services is, as D'Andra Millsap observes, "erratic at best." Estimates differ, but most suggest that only 70 percent of private insurers cover infertility treatment, and only 20 percent cover IVF.[4] About 40 percent of large self-insured employers include some form of advanced fertility services (e.g., fertility drug therapy with artificial insemination) in employee health benefit packages, but most exclude such treatments as IVF.[5] Thirteen U.S. states have enacted legislation requiring insurance carriers to cover or offer coverage for infertility, but what is covered varies widely: costs for diagnosis might be reimbursed but not costs for treatment, surgical correction and monitoring but not fertility drugs, hormonal or surgical treatment but not IVF. Moreover, mandated coverage laws do not apply to all employers. Small or self-insured companies and religious institutions, for example, are typically exempt from providing coverage for infertility services. With an average success rate of 25 to 35 percent per attempt and a price tag of between $7,000 and $10,000, it is not unusual for couples needing IVF to pay out $30,000 or more in the pursuit of a successful pregnancy.

In the United States, the exponential growth in the availability and use of sophisticated infertility services has coincided with the advent of managed care. Paradoxically, managed care restructuring has both increased and decreased the likelihood of insurance coverage for "high end" or advanced fertility therapies. Competition for contracts by managed care plans puts pressure on brokers to offer comprehensive, attractive benefit packages and on competitive companies to purchase them. Assisted reproduction in an affordable plan appeals to companies whose valued or vocal employees include those with the greatest investment in infertility services: upper-middle-class professional women.[6]

At the same time, as *New York Times* reporter Anne Adams Lang observed, in today's increasingly cost-conscious and cost-driven market, insurance carriers are "mostly like poltergeists haunting the field of reproductive medicine. They materialize with ephemeral policies that are changed or withdrawn in a flash."[7] The January 1998 announcement by Aetna, one of the country's largest insurers, that it was dropping in vitro fertilization from its U.S. Healthcare Plan and a similar announcement in June by Group Health, one of New York's largest insurers, illustrate exactly how quickly "fringe benefits" like infertility treatment become casualties when bottom line concerns lead to higher rates and pared benefits. Because Aetna was one of a relatively small number of companies offering coverage for IVF, too many women sought coverage with Aetna. The policy, according to a company spokesperson, was simply too expensive to continue.[8]

Several infertility-related measures have been introduced in Congress since 1998. The most recent is the Fair Access to Infertility Treatment and Hope Act of 2000 (S.R. 2160), introduced in March of 2000 by Sen. Robert Torricelli (D-NJ). If passed, it would require group health insurance plans across the country to provide benefits for the diagnosis and treatment of infertility, including four cycles of IVF.[9] Pointing to recent legal precedents as positive signs that the age of unquestioned exclusion for infertility treatment is coming to an end, lobbyists for the advocacy group Resolve and the American Society for Reproductive Medicine, an association of infertility specialists, are optimistic that even if the measures currently under consideration fail, a federal infertility mandate of some kind will eventually pass. The White House decision to require Medicaid coverage for Viagra, for example, opens the door for arguments for extending infertility coverage on sexual discrimination grounds. If treatment for male sexual dysfunction is "medically necessary," why not treatment for female infertility? A successful class-action suit against the city of Chicago in 1998 argued that denying infertility benefits violates the Americans with Disabilities Act.[10] And in a 1998 decision many advocates consider providential, the Supreme Court judged reproduction "a major life activity." Although the case concerned AIDS, the designation is valuable legal ammunition against the frequent claim that infertility, while disappointing, is not a *disease* nor a *disorder*.[11]

But efforts to secure state mandates for infertility coverage on the whole have been unsuccessful, and there is little reason to think that mandates will be any more popular on the federal level. When residents of Oregon were asked to prioritize health care services for Medicaid recipients, treatment for infertility came out at the bottom of the list. Identified as a "service valuable to certain individuals," infertility treatment was judged neither "essential" nor "very important" in light of community values.[12] In an unscientific but telling poll conducted on the Internet website "Parentsplace.com" in May of 1999, 80 percent of respondents answered "No" to the question: "Should insurance cover infertility treatment?"

It is difficult to know how to interpret such results, of course, without having access to information such as demographic profiles. In the case of the Oregon voters, it is difficult to separate the fate of infertility treatment from the context of the exercise—that is, the job of deciding health benefits for recipients of public assistance. Moreover, assessments of the importance of infertility shift when infertility is considered alone (where respondents tend to rank its importance highly) versus considered alongside other medical goods and services.[13] Still, taken as a fairly typical "knee-jerk" reaction, the overwhelmingly negative response to the question of guaranteeing access to infertility treatment reflects the depth of the resistance advocates face in attempting to expand coverage. Fertility is something we take for granted, but we are at a loss, when pressed, to isolate its precise value. Fertility has shifting social importance: in times of prosperity and plenty, it means something different than in times of struggle and scarcity. It also has multiple personal meanings. Having and raising children is a widely shared and highly prized human experience that many people quite comfortably forgo.

Whatever the outcome of current legal and legislative efforts on behalf of infertile patients, the debate over coverage for infertility treatment is not likely to end anytime soon, nor are the ethical issues at stake likely to become any less complex. The fight to secure access to infertility treatment in the United States is waged against the backdrop of an already over-inflated national health care budget and significant inequalities in access to basic health services. For many people, developing expensive technology for use on otherwise healthy people to address a problem that is as much social as medical epitomizes the mismatch between our contemporary appetite for technology and our ultimately limited economic resources. More than 40 million Americans in any calendar year lack adequate medical coverage, so providing expensive therapies for the one in seven American couples who are infertile seems a bit like air conditioning the top floor of a building that is on fire from the ground up. But access to infertility treatment is arguably also a matter of justice. Allowing carriers and employers to exclude advanced infertility treatment from medical insurance plans creates a two-tiered reproductive medicine system in which only the well-to-do have access to effective therapies. Those who cannot afford the costs of expensive fertility drugs or available methods of assisted reproduction are not just inconvenienced, they are denied the means to realize a basic and highly valued human good. Moreover, by ignoring infertility, insurers push assisted reproduction far into the for-profit medical market where treatment decisions are too often driven more by what a given patient wants and can afford than by the standards of good medicine.

Much has been written on the ethical questions raised by the new reproductive technologies.[14] Initial worries that "test tube" conception would endanger offspring, expressed so memorably by Protestant ethicist Paul Ramsey in the early days of IVF, have not been borne out.[15] To be sure, medically assisted reproduction is not risk-free. The tendency of IVF mothers to be older and to experience higher rates of multiple gestation results in increased incidence of pregnancy-related complications, premature birth, and caesarian section.[16] Recent studies raise questions regarding the impact of ICSI on early childhood development and long-range reproductive health. But there appears to be no material risk inherent in being conceived in a petri dish.[17] With more than 33,000 babies born since IVF was introduced in the United States, there is every reason to think that reproductive technologies can be used safely. Indeed, parenting through IVF hardly raises an eyebrow today. The once familiar "Brave New World" anxieties are now reserved for experiments at the envelope's edge—a successful birth through IVF in a sixty-two-year-old woman, a proposal for inserting human genetic material into cow eggs, or the discovery of a process for cloning a human being.

Hardly anyone today would call IVF "immoral experimentation on the unborn" as Ramsey had. But there is no doubt that these twenty-plus years of assisted reproduction represent a profound human experiment, the long-range risks, costs, and consequences of which are still unknown. Princeton molecular biologist Lee Silver is not exaggerating when he observes that the birth of the first IVF baby represented a "singular moment in human evolution," a moment in which it became possible "in a very literal sense . . . to hold the future of our species in our own hands."[18] Although developed for the treatment of infertility, IVF opens up possibilities for reproductive and genetic manipulations far beyond assisted reproduction. By "bringing the embryo out of the darkness of the womb and into the light of day," IVF allows for *and makes acceptable* manipulation of the embryo on the cellular level, the transfer of embryos from "one maternal venue to another," and the ability to access and alter genetic material.[19] Reproductive technologies invent new forms of parenting faster than we can find terms to describe them, raising questions about the nature of genetic property, the source and scope of parental obligations, and the limits of procreative liberty that we have only begun to face. The California case *Buzzanca v. Buzzanca*, which gave us, if only briefly, the first "parentless child," is just a hint at the conceptual revolution that is under way.[20] Moreover, the growth of fertility clinics in the United States has paralleled the bitter and intractable public debate over legalized abortion. It is not surprising, therefore, that there has been a great deal of attention given to the dangers of alienating reproduction from the body and the impact of assisted reproduction, particularly new forms of collaborative reproduction, on understandings of sexuality, reproduction, and parenthood. Neither is it surprising that the debate over the morality of assisted reproduction, particularly in theological circles, has often focused on the moral and legal status of the preembryo and the ethical quandaries that follow from the ability to manipulate embryonic life: What ethical norms should be adopted for the treatment of human embryos? Under what conditions and for what purposes is it ethical to create embryos or to destroy embryos?

Given the significance of reproduction in the lives of women and the ambiguous—often painful—history of women's experience with medical intervention in pregnancy and childbirth,[21] it is no wonder as well that reproductive and what are often called "reprogenetic" technologies have been a preoccupation for feminists and that the questions of women's agency and the social control of reproduction have held center stage. Feminists have not responded to the growth of reproductive technologies in a single voice. Indeed, in certain ways assisted reproduction has been a crucible issue, dividing feminists into camps and calling into question the coherence and self-definition of the emerging field of feminist ethics. If it was once clear to feminists what it meant to say that each woman should be able to determine for herself, freely and without penalty, the circumstances under which she will bear children, it is no longer so as the context shifts from access to safe contraception and abortion to IVF or commercial surrogacy. Feminists have always recognized that the disposition of the self in the event of reproduction, the choice that is most private and individual, is also what most intimately unites all women. Yet the infertile woman in the age of technology brings the complexities of this reality into stark relief. The woman who gives her body over to infertility specialists or purchases the reproductive services of another woman in pursuit of her reproductive interests (or needs or desires) redefines "a woman's right to choose" in a way that is perhaps ironic but at the very least has profound implications for the needs and interests of women everywhere.

There is no single "feminist position" on reproductive technologies. While some feminists have seen these technologies as valuable means of promoting women's reproductive liberty and addressing the acute suffering often associated with infertility, especially for women, others have expressed deep reservations about methods of reproduction that could leave women more rather than less vulnerable to exploitation. Some of the most vocal critics of reproductive technology have formed the Feminist International Network on Resistance to Reproductive and Genetic Engineering (FINRRAGE), which has lobbied heavily for an international ban on the development and clinical use of reproductive and reprogenetic technologies. Whatever else has divided feminists, however, they have been united in an acute sensitivity to issues of race, class, and gender in the assessment of technology, as well in an appreciation of the importance of bearing witness to the long and complex history of women's reproductive role within patriarchal society.

For all the attention to the social, political, and legal dimensions of reproductive technologies, however, the debate, both inside and outside of feminist contexts, has centered largely on the problem of assessing the meaning of intervention into the reproductive process. As a result, there has been very little substantive reflection on the questions of distributive justice raised by medically assisted reproduction. Concerns for justice in regard to assisted reproduction have most often been raised in order to clarify the rights and obligations of various parties in reproductive relationships.[22] Inequalities in access and the high cost of treatment are frequently mentioned in the table of ethical issues posed by assisted reproduction, and commentators have certainly staked positions on whether the inability to afford medical treatment for infertility is unfair or merely unfortunate.[23] But I know of no full-length work that attempts to offer a comprehensive, systematic, and theological analysis of the ethical questions at stake in arguments over access to assisted reproduction: What is the place of reproductive technologies in socially responsible medicine? Is a just society obligated to assist couples or individuals in their desire for biological offspring? Are problems such as infertility best understood as medical or social? What are the most useful mechanisms for measuring expenditures and outcomes with respect to reproductive medicine?

This book is such an attempt. It is an effort to reflect ethically and theologically on the experience of infertility and the economic, ethical, and political dimensions of reproductive medicine. Although I write as an infertile woman, having experienced firsthand what so many have called the "torturous roller coaster" of infertility treatment, what follows is not a personal account of infertility or an exercise in patient advocacy. I was a "typical" infertility patient—white, upper middle class, over thirty—but I cannot claim that my story is representative of the experience of infertility treatment in the United States. As a professional couple with two incomes and an insurance plan that provided good coverage for certain types of treatment, my husband and I were shielded from the full financial toll of infertility, but not from its emotional and relational toll. My aim is not to speak for the infertile in the debate over access to treatment, but to probe the serious and complex questions of justice prompted by the growth of reproductive medicine in the United States. At the same time, they are questions the shape and urgency of which I could not have understood nearly as well without having been a patient myself. As Paul Lauritzen showed so clearly in *Pursuing Parenthood,* some aspects of reproductive medicine are better understood from the inside, and moral analysis is enriched when objective claims, for example, about the exploitation of women under assisted reproduction, are tested against personal and reflexive experience.[24]

In the same way, although I will argue for a view of distributive justice in health care in which some claims to treatment for infertility can be justified, my goal is not primarily to defend a position on the rights of infertile patients to treatment or the duties of insurers to include IVF in a basic benefits package. Rather, I take debates over access to expensive, "last resort" therapies for infertility as a springboard to explore the fundamental questions posed by the challenge of setting health care goals and priorities in the face of expanding technological capabilities and growing economic constraints: How should we understand the relationship between individual wants, needs, and desires and the social or "common" good? How do we weigh the importance of "saving" lives versus "creating" lives, of life-prolonging versus life-enhancing medicine? How do working definitions of health and disability function in debates over access in particular societies? What is the proper role of political process (e.g., patient-group lobbying) in the assignment of health care priorities?

The presupposition of this book is that any attempt to answer such questions requires a satisfactory account of human flourishing. To articulate goals and priorities for medicine today, whether for reproductive medicine or medicine in general, requires that we attend adequately to the social dimension of personhood and the character of health as a capacity or power to participate in the common life. My analysis is influenced by contemporary feminist thought, particularly by efforts to articulate a vision for women's health that aims not just at the cure of disease but at the creation of social and political conditions for achieving and maintaining physical, emotional, and social well-being. It shares with feminist ethics a central interest in the dynamics of power (emotional and physical as well as social, political, and economic) that underlie professional-patient relationships and within which genuine moral agency in medical decision making is promoted or constrained. Although I disagree with those feminists who argue for a legislative ban on access to reproductive technologies, I share their concern regarding the implications of the medicalization of reproduction for women's reproductive agency. I reach different conclusions, but I take from their critique a necessary caution about the ambiguity of reproductive choice in a gendered society.

My analysis also draws from the modern tradition of Roman Catholic social thought. Relying on the relational anthropology of the U.S. Catholic bishops' pastoral letter on the economy (*Economic Justice for All*)[25] and papal encyclicals such as *Pacem in Terris, Sollicitudo Rei Socialis*, and *Centesimus Annus*,[26] I presuppose the intrinsic interrelation of individual agency and the common good. I presuppose, as well, a view of rights as "shares" in the minimum conditions of human well-being in society. Thus, it will not be enough to ask "How far should a society go to help individuals satisfy their interests in reproduction?" The prior question of social justice (within which questions of justice in health care must be set) is: "Under what conditions can material goods sufficient to meet the basic needs of all members be produced and fairly distributed, meaningful participation in the civic community made possible, and valued human pursuits (e.g., family life, education, artistic and cultural expression) supported?"

Finally, my analysis is influenced by Daniel Callahan's perceptive critique of contemporary Western medicine.[27] Callahan's views on health care rationing have been controversial. However, no one has more effectively unmasked the dangerous pretensions of our cure-oriented, death-denying health care system. Nor has anyone argued more persuasively for our need to face the growing gap between investments in medicine and achievements in health *care*. In the end, I give treatment for infertility a higher priority than would Callahan. But I take seriously his point that moral assessments of the means we choose for resolving infertility cannot be separated from open examination of the ends we seek, and the question of obligations or limits in assisted reproduction cannot be posed apart from the question of the goods and purposes that medicine should serve. I also share Callahan's aspirations for an American health care system that is "temperate, affordable, sustainable, and equitable."[28] Thus, although I will argue for a universal right to health care that includes some level of access to treatment for infertility, I do not suppose that medicine should serve all human desires nor that medicine is always the best healer. Rather, as Callahan argues in *The Troubled Dream of Life*, medicine's role is to alleviate the suffering brought about by failures of the body, to address the physical and psychological manifestations of the problems of human mortality. That is all it can do and that is all it should do.[29] The challenge, of course, is deciding what exactly medicine's contribution should be in the particular forms of suffering occasioned by infertility.

The argument I advance for the place of reproductive technologies in a "temperate, affordable, sustainable, and equitable" health care system unfolds in three broad steps. First, I will give a brief look at the economics of medically assisted reproduction in the United States. There is nothing especially original in the observation that disparities in access to infertility treatment in the United States pose questions of distributive justice. Nor is there anything especially new in the acknowledgment that problems of macro- and microallocation are among the most intractable problems for medical ethics. What is not obvious, however, is the degree to which current economic arrangements themselves create ethically questionable conditions in assisted reproduction. Chapter 1, therefore, uncovers three misconceptions that operate in existing patterns of funding for infertility. The purpose in starting here is to show how current strategies for containing the social costs or avoiding the social burden of assisted reproduction not only fail to be effective but have their own ethical consequences. Efforts to defer social debate over the value of assisted reproduction prove, on examination, to be both unsuccessful and costly. Thus, I argue that the fundamental questions of how to weigh assisted reproduction in a table of health care priorities cannot be avoided. More important, I show that facing the problem of limits requires a conceptual shift in the way we think about medically assisted reproduction. Only by ceasing to treat assisted reproduction as a luxury or consumer good do we bring it into the arena where questions of medical appropriateness and social responsibility are raised.

Next, I make the case that addressing infertility (even where it requires the use of high-tech therapies such as IVF) is defensible within a broad view of the purposes of medicine and a commitment to women's health.[30] Chapter 2 provides an overview of the ethical issues raised by assisted reproduction and a justification for at least some forms of assisted reproduction. Chapter 3 takes Eric Cassell's illuminating account of suffering as a starting point for articulating and justifying a professional responsibility to address infertility. Since what is ultimately at stake, however, is the place of assisted reproduction in socially responsible medicine, I also draw on the conclusions of the International Project on the Goals of Medicine, spearheaded by Callahan, to explore the importance of assisted reproduction in a comprehensive but temperate view of health and of the obligations of societies to sustain it.

Finally, I consider possibilities for bringing an ethic of restraint to bear on the development and use of medically assisted reproduction. Chapter 4 takes up the questions of procreative liberty that are central to debates over assisted reproduction, especially in the United States. Claims about the "sacred" status of procreative rights often function as trump cards, effectively foreclosing serious discussion of the social dimensions of reproductive decisions. Thus, any attempt to assess the limits of obligations to promote fertility must begin, as I do here, with a critique of prevailing, highly individualistic accounts of procreative liberty. Drawing in part from the Roman Catholic social tradition, I argue for a view of reproductive liberty that places the right to procreate within commitments to the common good. It treats reproduction as essentially social, and reproductive rights as inherently involving social and relational responsibilities. Both claims to treatment and their limits can be seen to follow from the nature of liberty (and procreative liberty) within an ethic of the common good.

Chapter 5 draws together the conclusions of chapters 2 and 3 in a modest argument for equitable access to assisted reproduction for the infertile. Here I take up directly the questions of how we might weigh the importance of assisted reproduction against other social and medical goods and where we might draw the line in social obligations to promote fertility. I rely in small part on the capabilities account being developed by philosophers such as Martha Nussbaum to fill out my account of the obligations of distributive justice. I argue, therefore, for access to assisted reproduction as a means of protecting an important aspect of social participation, particularly for women. At the same time, I acknowledge that how far obligations extend is a matter of a particular society's abilities to ensure even more basic or fundamental aspects.

The final chapter explores questions of faith and infertility. It has become clear in the debate over assisted suicide in the United States that religious communities must do more than simply articulate the morally unaccept-able options for the dying. Rather, if the dying and those who care for them are to resist what is held to be the death-denying choice of assisted suicide, they require the care of the community and the full resources of an honest and aware faith. If we are to recognize moral limits to what we may do to relieve suffering, then we have also, as faith communities, to teach people how to live with integrity and how to die well within those limits. Although there are ob-vious differences between terminal illness and infertility, the lesson of assisted suicide is important: If we are to acknowledge limits (either moral or practi-cal) to what we may do to relieve the suffering associated with infertility, then we must articulate a compassionate spirituality for the infertile. We must, in other words, develop resources within the liturgical and pastoral life of the church for living within the limits of involuntary childlessness with hope and dignity. Drawing from the story of the hemorrhaging woman in the Gospel of Luke, I offer a reflection on the possibilities for developing a theology of ac-ceptance in the face of the death of dreams and expectations that marks the ex-perience of infertility.

A final note. Marsh and Ronner observe that childlessness was seldom discussed by women writers before the twentieth century and almost never by men. One exception was Henry Adams, who was said to have anguished over his childless marriage. In the face of yet another birth announcement by a friend, he writes: "I wish . . . [I] wish . . . that the mystery of Birth and the Grave were either less important to us, or more encouraging."[31] Throughout this book, I have tried to remain attentive to the intense importance of child-bearing, especially for those who are unable to realize it without assistance. Although fertility has various meanings and values as a social reality, prob-lems of infertility are experienced for a great many people as a clear, unam-biguous sorrow. A commitment to the common good means that the alleviation of individual suffering or the satisfaction of individual desires cannot be inde-pendent or isolated values. Still, I have tried to remind us along the way that wherever we draw the lines, we ought not forget that the mysteries of which we speak are not, by difficulty or decision, made any less important to those who find themselves on the wrong side of them.

NOTES

1 National success rates for 1997 (the latest year for which data are available) are 27.7 percent for IVF, 29.9 percent for gamete intrafallopian transfer (GIFT), and 28 percent for zygote intrafallopian transfer (ZIFT). For women over 39 the overall success rate for IVF and IVF-related therapies is 13 percent. Centers using day 5 blastocyst transfers report rates of 50 to 60 percent. Success rates for donor egg programs nationally are approximately 40 percent. Information provided by the Centers for Disease Control [http://www.cdc.gov/nccdphp/drh/index.htm].

2 Michael Lemonick, "The New Revolution in Making Babies," *Time* (December 1, 1997), 42.

3 Tamara L. Callahan, Janet E. Hall, Susan L. Ettner, Cindy L. Christiansen, Michael F. Greene, William F. Crowley, Jr., "The Economic Impact of Multiple-Gestation Pregnancies and the Contribution of Assisted-Reproduction Techniques to Their Incidence," *New England Journal of Medicine* 331, no. 4 (July 28, 1994): 244–49.

4 D'Andra Millsap, "Sex, Lies, and Health Insurance: Employer-Provided Health Insurance Coverage of Abortion and Infertility Services and the ADA," *American Journal of Law and Medicine* 23, no. 1 (1996): 57.

5 Source: A. Foster Higgins and Co., a benefits consulting firm. Nineteen percent of HMOs offer coverage for in vitro fertilization. Source: The William Mercer Companies, "Aetna Cuts Its Coverage for Advanced Fertility Care," *New York Times* (January 10, 1998), A8.

6 Sarita Russ Gocial, "The Infertility Practice: Managed Care," *International Journal of Fertility* 40, no. 3 (1995): 118–19.

7 Anne Adams Lang, "For Infertility Treatments, Now You're Covered, Now You're Not," *New York Times* (June 21, 1998), 12.

8 Milt Freudenheim, "Aetna Is Reducing Fertility Benefits," *New York Times* (January 10, 1998), A8.

9 "Bills to Expand Infertility Insurance Introduced, Vetoed," *The Guttmacher Report on Public Policy*, 3, no. 2 (April 2000) [http://www.agi-usa.org/pubs/journals/gr030213b.html]. Also pending at the time this book went to press: H.R. 2774, sponsored by Representative Marty Meehan (D-MA), requires federal employees' health plans to include coverage of infertility services; H.R. 2706, sponsored by Representative Anthony Weiner (D-NY), requires all health plans to include coverage for infertility services. Source: Resolve, Advocacy Updates [http://www.resolve.org/advitr1.htm].

10 *Bielicki v. City of Chicago*, 1997 U.S. Dist. Lexis 6880 (N.D. Ill. 1997).

11 *Abbott v. Bragdon*, 524 US 624 (1998).

12 See Charles J. Dougherty, "Setting Health Care Priorities: Oregon's Next Steps," *Hastings Center Report* 21, no. 3 (May–June 1991), supplement, 1–10. Other services in that category included treatment for diaper rash and viral warts.

13 Peter J. Neumann, "Should Health Insurance Cover IVF? Issues and Options," *Journal of Health Politics, Policy and Law* 22, no. 5 (October 1997): 1224.

14 See, for example, Paul Lauritzen, *Pursuing Parenthood: Ethical Issues in Assisted Reproduction* (Bloomington: Indiana University Press, 1993); Lori Andrews, *The Clone Age: Adventures in the New World of Reproductive Technology* (New York: Henry Holt, 1999); Irina Pollard, *A Guide to Reproduction: Social Issues and Human Concerns* (Cambridge: Cambridge University Press, 1994); Kenneth Alpert, ed., *The Ethics of Reproduction Technology* (New York: Oxford University Press, 1996); Lynda Beck Fenwick, *Private Choices, Public Consequences: Reproductive Technology and the New Ethics of Conception, Pregnancy and Family* (New York: Dutton, 1998).

15 Paul Ramsey, "On in Vitro Fertilization, Testimony on in Vitro Fertilization before the Ethics Advisory Board, Department of Health, Education and Welfare," reprinted in *On Moral Medicine: Theological Perspectives in Medical Ethics*, Stephen E. Lammers and Allen Verhey, eds. (Grand Rapids, Mich.: William B. Eerdmans Publishing Co., 1987), 340 [paraphrase].

16 Joseph G. Schenker and Yossef Ezra, "Complications of Assisted Reproductive Techniques," *Fertility and Sterility* 61, no. 3 (1994): 411–22.

17 Questions remain as to whether controlled ovarian hyperstimulation (COH), a standard protocol for infertility treatment, is safe for women. Although the data are inconclusive, concerns have been raised about whether

the medications used for COH pose long-range elevated risks of ovarian and breast cancer. The point here is simply that there is no greater incidence of birth defect associated with IVF than found in the general population.

18 Lee M. Silver, *Remaking Eden: Cloning and Beyond in a Brave New World* (New York: Avon Books, 1997), 75.

19 Ibid.

20 Jaycee was conceived via anonymous embryo donation transferred to a gestational surrogate. One month before delivery, John Buzzanca filed for dissolution of the marriage and asserted that he would bear no financial responsibility for the child. Citing the Uniform Parentage Act, the trial court found that no named party (John Buzzanca, his now ex-wife Luanne Buzzanca, or the gestational surrogate) could be the parent of Jaycee. On appeal, the California Court of Appeal for the 4th Appellate District ruled that the intended parents, John and Luanne Buzzanca, are the legal parents of Jaycee. *Buzzanca v. Buzzanca,* Sup. Ct. No. 95 D002992 (1998).

21 See Barbara Ehrenreich and Deidre English, *For Her Own Good: 150 Years of the Experts' Advice to Women* (New York: Doubleday/Anchor, 1978).

22 See Teresa Iglesias, *IVF and Justice: Moral, Social and Legal Issues Related to Human in Vitro Fertilisation* (London: The Linacre Center, 1990). See also LeRoy Walters's 1987 study of international committee statements on the ethical issues in reproductive technology, "Biomedical Ethics: A Multinational View," *Hastings Center Report* 17, no. 3 (June 1987): 1. For an exception, see Peter J. Neumann, "Should Health Insurance Cover IVF? Issues and Options," 1215–39.

23 For a fine treatment of distributive justice questions in assisted reproduction, see Patricia Beattie Jung, "What Price Fertility?" in *Infertility: A Crossroad of Faith, Medicine and Technology*, edited by Kevin W. Wildes, S.J. (Dordrecht: Kluwer Academic Publishers, 1997), 167–80.

24 Lauritzen, *Pursuing Parenthood.*

25 National Conference of Catholic Bishops, *Economic Justice for All: Pastoral Letter on Catholic Social Teaching and the United States Economy.* (Washington, D.C.: United States Catholic Conference, 1986).

26 *Pacem in Terris: Encyclical Letter of Pope John XXIII,* April 11, 1963 (Washington, D.C.: National Catholic Welfare Conference, 1963); *On Social Concern: Sollicitudo Rei Socialis, Encyclical Letter of Pope John Paul II,* December 30, 1987 (Washington, D.C.: United States Catholic Conference, 1988); On the hundredth anniversary of *Rerum Novarum: Centesimus Annus*, addressed by the Supreme Pontiff Pope John Paul II (Washington, D.C.: United States Catholic Conference, 1991).

27 See Daniel Callahan, *The Troubled Dream of Life: Living with Mortality* (New York: Simon and Schuster, 1993); *What Kind of Life? The Limits of*

Medical Progress (New York: Simon and Schuster, 1990); also, symposium honoring Callahan's contribution to bioethics, *Hastings Center Report* 26, no. 6 (November–December 1996).

28 I take this description from the coda of the report of the Hastings Center project on the goals of medicine. See "The Goals of Medicine: Setting New Priorities," *Hastings Center Report* 26, no. 6 (November–December 1996): S26.

29 Callahan, *The Troubled Dream of Life*, 101.

30 "The Goals of Medicine: Setting New Priorities," Special Supplement, *Hastings Center Report* 26, no. 6 (November–December 1996): S9.

31 Marsh and Ronner, *The Empty Cradle,* 100.

CHAPTER ONE

THE ECONOMICS OF INFERTILITY

Pergonal n. bankruptcy in injectable form.

In late November of 1997, the national media's attention was riveted on a small Iowa town, where a 29-year-old mother of one, the wife of a billing clerk at the local Chevrolet dealership, had just given birth to septuplets. The McCaughey babies were quickly dubbed "the Miraculous Seven," their against-the-odds survival touted as a testament to modern medicine, old-fashioned faith, and simple good luck. But not everyone viewed the event as a cause for celebration. Bobbi McCaughey's refusal to consider selective reduction (a procedure in which one or more fetuses in a multiple pregnancy are aborted to improve the chances of a healthy birth for those remaining) was called foolish and irresponsible. The fact that powerful fertility drugs like the Metrodin that Bobbi McCaughey took can be prescribed by any general practitioner or obsetrician-gynecologist (OB-GYN) was repeatedly cited as evidence of the virtually unregulated "Wild West" state of reproductive medicine in the United States. And even for the romantic, the approximately $40,000 per baby price tag was a stark reminder of the rising social costs of assisted reproduction.[1]

Many fertility experts find the national fascination with multiple births dangerous. Media hype of the sort that followed the arrival of the McCaughey babies and, soon after, the birth of octuplets to Nkwm Chukwu of Texas distorts public perceptions about the state of infertility treatment, making exceptional cases into the norm. While news reports are quick to point out that new drug therapies and IVF technologies account for a rising rate of multiple births, they are slower to admit that successful treatment ends in a single birth most of the time. Media attention of this sort is no great gift to patients who already feel as though they have to justify their pursuit of parenthood and to a medical specialty that often finds itself on the defensive. Even more serious, national celebrations of "miraculous" births like the McCaughey septuplets mask the difficulties and risks involved in multiple gestation pregnancies. As Dr. Alan Copperman, director of Reproductive Endocrinology at Mt. Sinai–New York University Medical Center in New York observed, "it seems there is almost an acceptance these days of quads or quints or even more, and the outrage gets less and less as we hear about more and more of these cases. The fact is that the vast majority of these cases end in disaster, sometimes for the mom, most often for the babies." According to fertility specialists such as Copperman, by focusing only on the successes, media attention creates false security: "Every time a case comes along like that of Ms. Chukwu or Bobbi McCaughey . . . some desperate couples become more willing to take greater risks. It's almost like an arms race."[2]

The public debate generated by the McCaughey or Chukwu sensations does serve, however, to surface certain popular misconceptions about the costs of infertility and assisted reproduction. Examining them is useful in showing not only how the economic and the ethical *intersect* in reproductive medicine but how, to some degree, the economic *structures* the ethical.

Myths and Realities in the Economics of Infertility

Myth #1: IVF Accounts for the High Cost of Infertility Treatment

Released in the fall of 1993, the Clinton Health Security Plan was a first-pass (and ultimately failed) attempt to address the growing cry for health care reform in the United States. It promised "comprehensive health coverage . . . regardless of health or employment status" in a managed care, managed competition delivery system.[3] Among its many ambitions, the plan attempted to sketch the dimensions of a "guaranteed national benefits package." As described in the draft report of September 7, 1993, the proposed package included hospital services, emergency care, clinical preventive services, physical therapy, and treatment for mental illness. It did not include

> *services that are not medically necessary and appropriate, private duty nursing, cosmetic orthodontia and other cosmetic surgery, hearing aids, adult eyeglasses and contact lenses, in vitro fertilization, sex change surgery and related services, private room accommodations, custodial care, personal comfort services and supplies and investigational treatments. . . .[4]*

The Clinton plan's comprehensive benefits package did not exclude treatment for *infertility*. Indeed, lobbyists for Resolve and the American Society for Reproductive Medicine (then the American Fertility Society) were assured that infertility would be included in the working table of health care needs. But the inclusion of IVF among the list of "medically unnecessary" and "luxury services" made good on the warning they also received that IVF would be excluded from the table.

The Clinton plan's exclusion of IVF from a guaranteed benefits package is representative of reimbursement patterns in general. Outside of the few states where insurance carriers are required to cover IVF, infertility treatment, when it is covered at all, is generally limited to diagnosis or "diagnosis and treatment of correctable medical conditions."[5] Insurers have justified exclusion of IVF on several grounds: (1) infertility is not an illness; (2) IVF is not medically indicated because it does not correct the underlying medical problem; and (3) IVF is an experimental therapy.[6] All of these grounds have been contested. Efforts to deny coverage for IVF on the grounds that infertility is not an illness have been criticized as arbitrary and inconsistent.[7] Since the majority of carriers cover at least some infertility services (e.g., diagnostic tests and procedures or surgical correction of endometriosis), to exclude IVF on these grounds results, not in excluding infertility as an illness category, but in treating only some forms of infertility as illness. Moreover, insurers typically employ a broad understanding of illness, including as "diseases" conditions such as "chemical dependency, congenital defect of a child's soft palate, alcoholism, hernias, headaches, senility, exogenous obesity and insanity caused by syphilis."[8] If some notion of "impaired bodily function" or "loss of physical or emotional capacity" defines insurers' ordinary practice, as it arguably does, the exclusion of many forms of infertility from the category of "illness" (e.g., scarred or missing fallopian tubes) appears inconsistent or dependent on a capriciously narrow understanding of "illness."

At first blush, the exclusion of IVF on the grounds that it will not cure infertility seems to rest on a firmer rationale. It is true that IVF merely circumvents the problem of impaired fertility. Indeed, in some instances, IVF is performed on healthy, "fertile" patients, for example, in order to overcome infertility that follows from a sperm problem. But, as the court argued in *Ralston v. Connecticut General Life Insurance Company*, excluding a treatment on the grounds that it does not cure an underlying medical problem "does not accord with reason, common sense, or the ordinary practice within the insurance industry."[9] Applied consistently, this rationale would entail refusing coverage for any condition for which there exists "no known cure." Setting aside whatever problems might be involved in instituting such a principle of exclusion for determining health benefits, the fact is, as the court noted, evidence that a proposed treatment will *cure* an underlying medical problem is not now ordinarily required as a standard of inclusion. What is required is evidence that the treatment works as well or better than presently available methods. Moreover, as was argued in a similar case, consistent application of this principle would require denying coverage for any treatment that merely compensates for or replaces a lost or impaired bodily function, for example, kidney dialysis, coronary by-pass surgery, limb prosthesis, and the insulin pump.[10]

The argument that IVF is experimental is also initially persuasive. IVF technologies have only been in wide clinical use for twenty-five years and have developed along a fairly sharp learning curve. Although much is now known about the conditions for successful fertilization and embryo development in vitro, relatively little is understood concerning conditions affecting success or failure at the implantation stage. Thus, developments in treatment have had an inescapably experimental or trial-and-error character. Even when IVF results in a successful pregnancy, clinicians cannot always explain why. More important for present purposes, success rates for IVF have long hovered at 25 to 35 percent. In a 1988 case, *Reilly v. Blue Cross and Blue Shield United*, the trial court accepted the insurer's argument that a treatment with success rates of under 50 percent could be considered experimental.[11]

But here again the invocation of this rationale for IVF exclusion requires a narrow and somewhat idiosyncratic use of "experimental." If a similar success rate of over 50 percent were required routinely as a standard for inclusion, nonpalliative treatment for the terminally ill would have to be excluded since treatment in such cases has a zero success rate.[12] Even if one were to grant a normative relation between low success rates and the designation "experimental," in fact the working meaning of the term in this context connotes "not yet customary use," that is, a therapy has not reached a level of safety and demonstrated efficacy so as to be generally accepted for clinical application. As we noted in the introduction, after the birth of more than 33,000 babies in the United States alone, it hardly seems accurate to continue to call IVF "experimental."[13]

Even a cursory look at typical reasons given by insurers for excluding IVF, even from infertility coverage, reveals them to be weaker, more transparent, than they seem at first hearing. Not surprisingly, what really drives efforts to jettison IVF (as well as the tendency not to question exclusion) is a raw perception of its cost and its dispensability. Underneath all rationales lies Aetna's simple—and seemingly self-evident—defense: Too many women wanted IVF and it was too expensive.[14]

One of the most persistent and pervasive myths concerning the costs of treating infertility is that IVF is a *uniquely* expensive response to infertility, and therefore that the costs of treating infertility can be controlled simply by excluding IVF. For the approximately 70 percent of traditional insurance carriers that offer at least some coverage for infertility, however, jettisoning IVF results in a more superficial and illusory cost-control than meets the eye. It is true that IVF and IVF-related therapies (e.g., gamete intrafallopian transfer

[GIFT], zygote intrafallopian transfer [ZIFT], and IVF with intracytoplasmic sperm injection [ICSI]) are expensive. Although costs vary depending on the type of therapy and the specific needs of the patient, average charges for IVF are, as we have seen, between $8,000 and $10,000 per completed cycle. This compares to $350 for an unmedicated intrauterine insemination (IUI). If we look just at the price tag, IVF looks obviously more expensive.

However, although the use of high-tech, expensive procedures is increasing,[15] most couples seeking treatment for infertility require only low-tech assistance. Even recent estimates suggest that only about 1 percent of infertility patients use IVF or IVF-related therapies.[16] Moreover, for some patients, early recourse to IVF would be less expensive and more cost-effective than recourse to conventional or low-tech methods. For women with tubal disease, for example, or in cases of male factor infertility, studies show that IVF is more effective and cheaper than conventional surgical methods.[17] For many older women, IVF also proves less expensive and at least as effective as long-term treatment with fertility drugs and IUI. Even more important, except for the most rudimentary of low-tech therapies, (such as, monitoring of ovulation by temperature changes), infertility treatment is often expensive long before recourse to IVF and IVF-related therapies. In a 1988 study on the medical and social aspects of infertility, the U.S. Office of Technology Assessment (OTA) estimated the total infertility expenditures nationally for 1987 at $1.0 billion. Of that amount, $66 million were classified as "IVF expenditures" while $935 million were "non-IVF expenditures."[18] To get a cost-breakdown for purposes of comparison, OTA divided infertility treatment into four typical stages: diagnosis and fertility drug treatment; complete evaluation of both partners; tubal surgery; and in vitro fertilization. The average cost of first-stage treatment was $3,668; second stage, $2,055; third stage, $7,118; and fourth stage, $9,376. Thus, comprehensive treatment for a woman with a fallopian tube obstruction could cost in the neighborhood of $13,000 without recourse to IVF and $22,217 with unsuccessful surgery and two cycles of IVF.[19] Current comparisons would have to take account of the higher utilization of IVF and IVF-related services. However, OTA's breakdown nicely illustrates the point that excluding expenditures for IVF does not automatically translate into low expenditures for the treatment of infertility.[20]

Some of the public perception about the high costs of IVF results from the association between IVF and rising rates of multiple gestation pregnancies. A 1994 study in the *New England Journal of Medicine* demonstrated the link between assisted reproduction and the incidence of multiple births: Of 13,206 births at the study hospital between 1986 and 1991, assisted reproduction was used in 2 percent of singleton births, 35 percent of twin births, and 77 percent of higher-order multiple gestations (e.g., triplets and higher).[21] The study also underscored the economic impact of multiple-gestation pregnancies. In 1991, hospital charges for a singleton birth were $9,845, as compared with $37,947 for twins, and $109,765 for triplets. "If all the multiple gestations resulting from assisted reproductive techniques had been single pregnancies," the researchers concluded, "the predicted savings to the health care delivery system in the study hospital alone would have been over $3 million per year."[22]

The practice of transferring more than one embryo in IVF accounts in part for the relationship between assisted reproduction and the increasing incidence of multiple births. The higher risks of prematurity and both maternal and neonatal complications associated with higher-order multiple births, as well as the significantly higher risks of perinatal mortality, raise serious medical and ethical questions, as well as economic questions, for assisted reproduction. But the risk of multiple gestation pregnancy is not confined to IVF, as both the McCaughey and Chukwu cases attest. The incidence of multiple gestation pregnancies ranges from 10 to 15 percent with the use of gonadotropins alone (i.e., "fertility" drugs, or injectable forms of the hormones used to stimulate the ovaries to produce eggs); 15 to 20 percent when gonadotropins are used with intrauterine insemination; and 15 to 30 percent with in vitro fertilization.[23] In each case, the risk of multiple gestation pregnancy is significant. However, the risk of multiple gestation with in vitro fertilization is only marginally greater than with the use of gonadotropins in combination with intrauterine insemination (IUI). Moreover, in principle, IVF affords a greater degree of control over the conditions for implantation than treatments using fertility drugs alone or fertility drugs in combination with IUI. In the latter case, once ovulation is stimulated and sperm is introduced, there is no way to prevent multiple implantation. In IVF, the clinician can choose how many or few embryos to transfer. In the wake of the McCaughey and Chukwu births, many fertility specialists noted that, in cases where ongoing monitoring suggested a high potential for multiple gestation pregnancy in a young woman undergoing drug therapy or drug therapy with IUI, responsible practice would be to cancel the cycle or convert to IVF. For reasons that we will explore later, "responsible practice" does not necessarily characterize the infertility industry as a whole or decisions concerning the transfer of embryos. Here the point is only that the problem of paying for multiple births cannot be avoided simply by jettisoning IVF.

Public perception of the uniquely high cost of IVF is also related, to some degree, to perceptions about costs versus outcomes. A widely reported and frequently cited study by Peter Neumann, Soheyla Gharib, and Milton Weinstein estimated the price tag for a single successful birth through IVF at between $50,000 and $800,000.[24] Defining "marginal cost per delivery" as "the cost incurred for a given cycle divided by the probability of achieving a delivery as a result of that cycle," they argued that a successful birth for a woman with the best chances of success (e.g., a young woman with tubal disease) costs $50,000 per delivery for the first cycle and $72,727 for the sixth cycle; for a woman with the worst chances (e.g., in a case involving male factor infertility) the cost was figured at $160,000 for the first cycle, rising to $800,000 in the sixth.[25] Several objections to the study's findings were raised: researchers used outdated figures and therefore underestimated chances of success while overestimating the number of times patients in a particular class would be likely to attempt IVF. Moreover, the use of estimated rather than actual costs gave a skewed picture of the expense of IVF. But the appeal of the study's conclusions, the frequency with which the $800,000 price tag is invoked in defense of excluding IVF from insurance coverage, makes it clear that Neumann and his colleagues struck a chord: The difficulty of achieving success with IVF joins with its high base price to create an image of IVF as financial quicksand.

The problem of weighing costs and outcomes in assisted reproduction is crucial, as we will see below. But an adequate cost-benefit analysis would have to include comparison between assisted reproduction and conventional methods of treating infertility. Some assessment of the possibilities for overcoming obstacles to successful assisted reproduction or lowering costs would be needed as well in order to separate costs associated with the development of a technology from costs intrinsic to a technology. Moreover, social costs of a treatment depend upon how that treatment is likely to be used and how costs will be distributed across populations. When Griffin and Panak studied the actual costs of providing coverage for infertility, including IVF, under Massachusetts' mandate for group plans, the increase in annual premium per person ($1.71 per month) was considerably lower than the $800,000 price tag would suggest.[26]

But what is finally problematic about arguments for IVF exclusion that rest on cost-benefit assumptions is that they presuppose a willingness to apply standards of allocation in the case of some forms of infertility that we are not willing to apply to the distribution of health care generally. Even where we grant the relevancy of weighing the costs versus benefits of a particular therapy in the determination of health care priorities, as we are increasingly forced to do in our current managed care climate, for most people cost-effectiveness is not the only or even the determinative value at stake. Indeed, a frequent criticism of managed care corporations is their willingness to sacrifice values such as relief of suffering, respect for dignity and patient autonomy, and fidelity between patient and provider for the sake of cost-effectiveness. In addition, policy decisions regarding the relative value of a particular therapy presume some level of public consensus on the appropriate goals of medicine.[27] They presume that we have some general idea of what ends are worth pursuing and what we want and can afford to spend in their pursuit. We have no such consensus in the United States at the present time.

The perception that IVF is a *uniquely* expensive response to infertility is powerful and widespread. Invoking the cost of IVF is often the magic bullet in defeating lobbying efforts by groups such as Resolve. But closer examination shows that it is more difficult than it appears to separate expenditures for IVF from expenditures for other infertility treatments, as well as to isolate the grounds on which we exclude infertility as a health-care benefit from the grounds on which we include other conditions. One consequence of treating IVF as a special case is a continued arbitrariness and incoherence in our treatment of infertility as a health care claim. A more serious consequence, as we will see, is that we risk, on the one hand, falsely privatizing IVF, and on the other hand, exempting other forms of infertility treatment from considerations of appropriateness, cost, effectiveness, and safety.

Myth #2: Assisted Reproduction Is a Private Matter

Assisted reproduction in the United States is largely a fee-for-service, private-market business. Because most insurance companies offer only partial coverage or none at all, patient share of costs for IVF and IVF-related therapies averages about 85 percent. This compares with a patient share of costs for IVF and IVF-related therapies of about 7 percent in France and 15 to 28 percent in Canada.[28] One consequence of high costs and little coverage is that access to assisted reproduction is determined principally by financial status. Some clinics limit access to IVF to married couples using their own gametes or women under forty, and some exclude single women and gay or lesbian couples. But in general, the type and extent of treatment—even whether one will be treated at all—are governed by how much the patient is able and willing to pay—usually, up front. As a result, there is a marked disparity between the epidemiological profile of infertile women in the United States (who are likely to be under 30, African American, with a high school education and a low income) and the profile of those receiving infertility services (who are typically over 30, white, middle class, with an average of two and one-half years of college). Despite the fact that married black women have an infertility rate one and one-half times higher than that of married white women, they represent a small percentage of infertility patients.[29]

There is another, less obvious consequence. Distributed under a private-market exchange, assisted reproduction—particularly with respect to high-end therapies such as IVF—functions conceptually as much like a consumer good as a medical good. Although subjected to media scrutiny, treatment decisions in medically assisted reproduction tend to escape the oversight to which other medical decisions are naturally subjected in a third-party payer system. More important, as a consumer good, assisted reproduction escapes the assumptions ordinarily at work in the distribution of medical goods, for example, that while a particular patient's well-being is paramount, other interests—social, institutional, professional—are also implicated; that health care is not simply a commodity but a service to individuals and communities; and that medical indications intersect with patients' wishes in the choice of appropriate treatment. This is not to say that infertility medicine operates outside of professional oversight; on the contrary, criticism of medically assisted reproduction has motivated professional societies such as the American Society for Reproductive Medicine to be vigilant in developing mechanisms for self-regulation. But treating assisted reproduction as a luxury item creates a climate in which the governing expectations are more like those in an ordinary retail exchange than in the usual delivery and receipt of medical care. Thus, it is not unusual to hear patients who have been discouraged from pursuing further attempts at IVF complain that the infertility specialist "has no right" to advise them not to go on, much less to refuse to perform another procedure. After all, they are paying the vast sums of money; whether or not a particular treatment is appropriate should be entirely up to them to decide.

In the background of such a response are common beliefs about economic privacy. In a liberal society we presume that individuals are free to spend their money however they wish—however foolishly or irresponsibly—so long as no one is materially harmed and minimum social obligations are met. If I want to spend $50,000 trying to conceive, it should be no one's business but my own, just as it would be no one's business if I spent $50,000 on a race car or a round-the-world cruise. But also intersecting with assumptions about the scope of economic liberty in this case are assumptions about the nature of reproductive liberty. It is taken for granted in the United States that individuals have a prima facie right to procreate, bear, and rear offspring without interference. Thus, how I go about pursuing parenthood, what medical or nonmedical means I use, and just as how much I spend, are nobody's business but my own.

It should be obvious by now that the line between public and private, personal resources and social resources, is not really so clear with regard to assisted reproduction. If a private insurer covers at least some forms of therapy for infertility—if, for example, fertility drugs like Pergonal and Metrodin are covered in a prescription drug plan—all payers and beneficiaries of that plan are, in some sense, sharing those costs. More important, since expenses for pregnancy and pregnancy-related conditions are generally covered in both public and private medical plans, the costs of a successful outcome are shared even if the expenses of infertility treatment are borne by individuals. This is especially significant when we take into account the high rate of multiple gestation pregnancies currently associated with medically assisted reproduction. Higher costs for obstetrical management, pre-delivery admissions, and intensive care nursery services are all implicated in multiple births, particularly in older women.[30] Long-term care for premature infants is extremely costly, often exceeding the parents' means (as in both the McCaughey and Chukwu cases). Simply in economic terms, assisted reproduction is not a private matter.

But one could argue that reproduction is never a purely private matter. Whether through reproductive technology or natural conception, bringing a child into the world is inherently *relational* (it always involves the establishment of a relationship between parent(s) and child) and inherently *social* (it always introduces into society a new member whose potential needs and capacities have social implications). Only by denying either the dependence of children or their ultimate independence is it possible to ignore the sense in which reproduction entails relational obligations. Indeed, one of the persistent criticisms of assisted reproduction (and our legal response to assisted reproduction) has been a tendency to define reproductive interests as though the wishes of procreators and the well-being of offspring could be isolated. As Daniel Callahan argued: "[I]t has been one of the enduring failures of the reproductive rights movement that it has, in the pursuit of parental discretion and the relief of infertility, constantly disassociated the needs of children and the desires of would-be parents."[31]

Even if we want to argue that there are good reasons to preserve a sphere of procreative liberty and to grant parents wide discretion in determining how to secure their children's best interests, we ought to acknowledge that the manner in which children are brought into the world is always a matter of social concern. The family has been assumed by many religions and cultures to be the primary or fundamental social unit. The stable, committed, "spousal" relationship is privileged as the fitting site for procreation, both because it is assumed that the well-being of children is—at least in general—best served under those conditions and because social stability is believed to be linked to familial stability. If there is any wisdom in these traditions, the potential of assisted reproduction to reconceive the family, possibly to alter our understanding of family irrevocably, argues against treating it as a private matter.

It is also significant that we are talking about *medically assisted* reproduction. Defenders of reproductive technologies are correct to resist the commonly invoked distinctions between *natural* and *unnatural* reproduction. Medical intervention into reproduction in itself does not render the process "unnatural", in the relevant sense of violating the laws of the body or perverting the natural order, any more than do other forms of medical intervention. But it is important to acknowledge the difference between procreation that can be accomplished without medical assistance and procreation that cannot be accomplished except with medical assistance. In the latter, the effort to reproduce implicates medicine, requires medical personnel, and uses medical resources. Just as it is appropriate to ask of any decision to put a patient on a mechanical ventilator whether this constitutes a right use of medical or social resources—questions that would be unnecessary could the patient breathe on her own—so it is appropriate to ask whether assisted reproduction in a given case constitutes a right use of medical and social resources. Given that society has a stake in responsible medical practice, decisions to reproduce that require medical assistance cannot be simply private decisions, not even to the degree that reproductive decisions can when they do not depend upon medical intervention. Moreover, because assisted reproduction aims ultimately at the birth of a child, issues of responsible practice extend to concerns for the health and well-being of potential offspring. In the wake of the Chukwu births, George Annas complained that "the ethics of the fertility industry [at present] focus exclusively on the interests of the couple who want to conceive. But the baby has to be considered here too. What responsibility does the medical community have to children who are born?"[32] Even if we disagree with his implicit indictment of the industry we can see why the question is not only reasonable but necessary.

It is, then, both the nature of reproduction and the character of reproductive technology that call into question the assumption that assisted reproduction is "nobody's business." Yet, insofar as we treat reproductive technologies as consumer or luxury goods, we place them outside the arena in which judgments of medical appropriateness and social responsibility are ordinarily made. Even worse, we create conditions that may actually encourage irresponsibility.

Myth #3: The Private Market Is the Best Means of Rationing IVF

Closely related to the myth that assisted reproduction is a private matter is the myth that social costs for assisted reproduction can be controlled or effectively shifted (to individuals) by leaving access up to the market. We have seen already how this belief functions in arguments for excluding IVF from medical benefits packages. We have seen already, as well, that the realities of cost-sharing for infertility treatment belie sharp distinctions between social and private, and the control of costs by jettisoning IVF may be much more illusory than the practice supposes.

But there are more serious problems with the assumption that free market forces will effectively control the costs of infertility treatment. Our experience with fee-for-service medicine in the United States has chastened expectations that health care costs will be moderated by the usual laws of supply and demand. Without intra- and extra-market controls, costs have tended to increase steadily such that overall spending for health care went from 5 percent of the gross national product (GNP) in 1950 to 15 percent in 1995. Certain features of the American health care system account for the high cost of care and the rapid growth in spending that ultimately generated the push for systemic restructuring in the early 1990s: high professional salaries, especially for specialty care; the tendency of third-party payment to insulate providers and patients from the true costs of care; defensive medicine and the high costs of malpractice insurance; rapid developments in medical technology; and institutional inefficiency.[33] But, as Gene Outka argues, there are also intrinsic features that make health care problematic as a market good. Assumptions that health care choices will (and should) respond to the values and principles of the market ignore the high importance of health care in individuals' lives and the relative vulnerability of the patient in the medical encounter. While we might walk away from a television that is too highly priced or comparison shop for one that is a better buy, most patients, particularly if they are in fear or physical distress, do not feel in a position either to assess for themselves the quality of their care or to forgo the more expensive in search of the cheaper.[34]

Increased availability of infertility services has not translated, generally speaking, into lower prices. Neither has the managed care revolution moderated costs in the infertility industry. Although capitation agreements can lower the prices insurers will pay for services considerably, the refusal of insurers to cover assisted reproduction leaves the prices of high-end services relatively untouched. The average charge for a single cycle of in vitro fertilization remains the same or more than it was in 1987.[35] Charges in the United States are the highest in the world; the base charge of $8,000 to $10,000 for IVF compares, for example, to U.S. $2,500 in Israel and between $1,000 and $1,500 in countries such as Belgium, Germany, and Greece.[36] Moreover, charges for assisted reproduction do not necessarily reflect costs. As one infertility specialist observes:

> *Assisted reproductive services represent relatively high fixed cost operations, yet both large and small programs in a given region have very similar charges. Why doesn't the high patient volume in larger programs lead to reduced charges? Why do gonadotropins manufactured in the same location by the same companies cost three to four times more in the United States than in other countries?*[37]

Infertility patients tend to be very well-educated medical consumers, often exchanging information via large Internet discussion lists. But as a patient group, an interest group, they are not well-organized politically. This is a factor, obviously, in the continued defeat in most states of insurance mandates for infertility treatment. It also accounts for a certain—and in ways surprising—powerlessness with respect to the infertility industry. Deeper than the vulnerability of the infertile as a group, however, is the vulnerability of individual patients. Infertile patients are certainly not in the position of the cancer patient; there is no fear of death or physical pain that compromises the willingness to walk away or demand a better price. But the intense, sometimes all-consuming desire for a child and, for older women in particular, the sense of limited time in which to find an answer, both motivates infertility patients to accept the high costs of treatment and makes them unwilling to "vote with their feet."

There is a more serious reason to question the assumption that the open marketplace is the best means for rationing IVF or controlling the social costs of infertility. In a surprisingly self-critical editorial in the professional journal *Fertility and Sterility,* Michael Soules, M.D., Director of the Division of Reproductive Endocrinology and Infertility at the University of Washington, identified several problems with current practices in infertility medicine. In general infertility care: (1) patients are often subjected to an extensive and prolonged series of tests with many duplications and overuse of diagnostic procedures such as laparoscopy; (2) there is an overuse of procedures that have a low chance of success (e.g., tubal reconstruction surgery); (3) conventional treatments are often extended beyond a reasonable duration of known efficacy; (4) these practices can extend over several years, often compromising the patient's best chances for achieving pregnancy. In assisted reproductive technology: (1) a lack of universal and enforceable safe practice guidelines creates wide disparities in standards, reported success rates, and risks of multiple birth; (2) the exclusion of assisted reproductive technologies from insurance coverage leads both patients and providers to choose more expensive but less efficacious treatment (e.g., tubal surgery over IVF); (3) competition between clinics and pressures for success by patients results too often in unsafe practices, such as the transfer of excessive numbers of embryos.[38]

There are several explanations for the problems Soules notes, including the fact that infertility is big business and there is a great deal of money to be made in dispensing infertility services. But, as he argues, "patients, physicians, government, and payers are all to blame" for overuse of noneffacacious treatment and, in particular, for practices that lead to a high rate of multiple births:

> *Patients, usually with limited financial resources, will accept the risk of multiple pregnancy because they can't afford the extra ART cycles necessary to achieve the same results with fewer embryos. Physicians are also responsible. . . . The competition between ART programs is intense; if a particular program voluntarily decreased the number of embryos transferred, the overall [pregnancy rate] inevitably would decrease. A drop in patient volume would follow. Although government intervention in the practice is not usually welcome or necessary, there is no government regulation pertaining to the number of embryos transferred as in other countries.[39]*

Soules points here to the subtle consequences of privatizing assisted reproduction. By treating reproductive technologies as a consumer good, making application and allocation responsive almost exclusively to retail market values, all parties—patients, professionals, payers, and government—participate in creating conditions under which, on the one hand, there are positive pressures toward irresponsible use of technology and, on the other, the absence of moderating pressures against ineffective or unacceptably risky treatment. We should be careful to avoid oversimplification here. The reasons for a largely "hands-off' approach to the regulation of assisted reproductive technologies in the United States are complex. As we noted earlier, there is a deep tradition of respecting reproductive privacy in this country as well as a tradition of self-regulation by the medical profession. In addition, the decision made in the 1980s to adopt a moratorium on federally funded embryo research has had the practical effect of isolating reproductive technologies from governmental oversight. But it is worth noting that many other countries (e.g., Germany, Australia, England, and Canada) have passed legislation regulating the practice of assisted reproduction, for example, limiting the number of embryos that can be transferred and restricting the use of gamete donors. In virtually every case, the government is the principle payer for assisted reproductive services.[40]

The effect of insurer oversight on clinical decision making is also complex and difficult to measure. One recent study, presented at the annual meeting of the American Society for Reproductive Medicine in October of 1998, showed a significantly lower rate of multiple births in states with the best insurance coverage as compared to those with little or no coverage. Researchers found, as they predicted, that both patients and physicians felt less pressure to transfer dangerously high numbers of embryos in states where further attempts would be covered. In addition, women with a high number of follicles (a condition that can also be a factor in multiple pregnancies) were more likely to forgo insemination where they were guaranteed another chance.[41] Currently, states with comprehensive coverage mandates also show lower success rates and thus a higher number of repeat attempts. To reduce overall costs, therefore, pressures to limit the number of embryos transferred would have to be accompanied by advances in predicting embryo quality. Recent success with blastocyst transfers (i.e., transfers of embryos at five days in vitro rather than three days) is promising in this regard. Since those embryos that survive to five days outside the body are more likely to continue to develop in utero, fewer can be transferred with better success rates.

We want to be very careful not to make naïve assumptions regarding the role of insurer oversight. But these studies are useful in showing how concerns for the cost-effectiveness of treatment and interests in standardizing practice guidelines, both inside and outside of reproductive medicine, arise in direct response to pressures by third-party payers to control the rising costs of care. All states having mandated coverage for infertility or Assisted Reproductive Technology also impose limits on services, either limits on the type of services covered or global limits on total expenditures. Regular processes of utilization review, however intrusive they may be in the eyes of physicians and patients, can provide an important context for accountability in treatment decisions. It is possible, in other words, for insurer oversight to exert a positive influence on the practice of assisted reproduction. Just to give one example of this potential: In January of 1999, Tufts Health Plan of Massachusetts announced that it would no longer pay for patients at three of nine fertility clinics in its system because the facilities did not meet minimum quality standards. The criteria included "rate of success, number of procedures done annually, number of physicians on the staff and how many are board certified, laboratory qualifications and 'patient-friendly' programs."[42] One of the clinics dropped by Tufts accused the insurer of manipulating data to avoid responsibility for providing coverage under Massachusetts' infertility mandate. But at least two of the others issued immediate statements announcing the steps they planned to take to comply with Tufts' criteria for reinstatement.

Intersection: Ethics and Economics

This brief look at common misconceptions about the economics of infertility should help us see, at least, that the interaction of the ethical and the economic in the context of medically assisted reproduction is more complex, the lines between public and private are less clear, and the strategies for containing the social costs or avoiding social responsibility for the burden of infertility care are less successful than our current practices suggest. However, showing that judgments concerning the status of assisted reproduction as a medical good are inconsistent and often arbitrary, does not take us very far in answering the central questions of this book. If the problem before us is "How are we to think about the care of the infertile in a health-care system that is 'temperate, affordable, sustainable, and equitable'" we cannot simply invoke inconsistencies or arbitrariness in current insurance practices. Cost containment strategies that allow treatment for some forms of infertility and not others or that presume too clear a demarcation between private and public expenditures may be capricious, shortsighted, or ultimately unwise, but it is not obvious that they are *unjust.* Only if we make certain assumptions about the character of assisted reproduction as a medical good, the nature of infertility as a disease or illness, and the meaning of "fairness" or "justice" in the distribution of health care would it also follow that such strategies are unfair or unjust. Whether existing disparities in access should be addressed as a matter of justice and if so, in what way, requires reflection on the nature of reproductive technologies and their place in an overall account of the purposes of medicine. We will take up this issue in the chapters that follow. For now, it is enough to see why the subject cannot be avoided, why deferring social debate over the value of assisted reproduction is both illusory and dangerous.

Distributive Justice and Assisted Reproduction

Today, announcements of "miraculous" developments in reproductive medicine coexist in the media with charges that the medical industry in the United States fails to treat persons justly and care for them well. To date, the United

States ranks first in the world in health care expenditures but remains sixteenth in the rate of infant mortality. Because of a steadily growing elderly population, the AIDS epidemic, rising health insurance premiums (leaving more people without health insurance or underinsured), cuts in Medicare, Medicaid, and Aid to Families with Dependent Children (AFDC) programs, and the continued high cost of treatment, the problems of access to health care nationally have become increasingly more acute in the last twenty years. Recent estimates suggest that upwards of forty million Americans are without health insurance at some point in every year, and the number of uninsured could grow to sixty million (or 24 percent of the population) by 2004.[43]

Until recently, the American medical system could be described as "primarily libertarian, with a safety net." That is, it was assumed that patients or in many cases, their employers, would pay for the level of care they desired and the necessary care of those who could not afford to pay would be subsidized, either by the state or by professional and institutional charity. There is no legally recognized "right" to health care in the United States. However, practices such as anti-dumping policies and cost shifting to cover indigent care reflected a working presumption that refusing life-saving care to those who cannot pay is ethically unacceptable. Pressures by employers to control the rising costs of health insurance made cost shifting increasingly difficult by the 1990s, giving new public urgency to the problem of access as well as to the problem of health care expenditures. Charles Dougherty suggests that "recent efforts at health care reform would not have been mounted had those concerned with financial issues not joined forces with those concerned about access." The failure of such efforts to result in a plan for universal coverage can be traced, he argues, to the "uneasy coalition of these two groups, especially to the reluctance of big business to accept a solution to its health care cost problems that involves a strong role for the federal government."[44]

The dramatic changes brought about by managed care restructuring have moved cost-consciousness into the heart of clinical decision making. However, as Karen Gervais and her coauthors note, very little has happened in the way of systemic reform. "The turn to managed care was a response to the cost-containment interests of purchasers. It was a change neither inspired by, nor organized to attain, crucial societal health care goals."[45] In for-profit managed care, in particular, there is little incentive to expand access to health care or to meet the health-related needs of those without coverage and little incentive to support professional training, research, and health education. Indeed, our relatively short experience with managed care in the United States has left many people doubtful that an unregulated medical marketplace will preserve even minimally responsible medicine, let alone generate a socially responsive health care system. "The market may give rise to 'healthy' competition," argue Gervais et al., "but it is unclear that it can give rise to healthy cooperation in relation to a communal good such as health care. Government-sponsored activity or regulation may be necessary to address and correct the unhealthy outcomes of market competition where the provision of this communal good is either not promoted or perhaps even undermined."[46]

The failure of health care reform is the backdrop against which questions of distributive justice in reproductive medicine today must be posed. It is no longer even practical to treat health care decisions as if they occur in a vacuum. The economic implications of clinical delusions have become transparent in a way they were not under the old fee-for-service arrangements and the inescapable limits on expenditures have shifted from the margins to the center of professional and public consciousness.[47]

One set of ethical questions we are now facing concerns the extent to which cost-containment measures should affect treatment decisions. A strict interpretation of the fiduciary responsibilities of the physician holds that economic considerations should never enter into judgments about initiating or continuing treatment. Increasingly, however, the decisional matrix in bioethics is shifting from physician-patient (or physician-patient-family) to physician-patient-society (or physician-patient-institution). While the physician's role as advocate for the medical interests of the patient remains primary, other interests (e.g., social interests in the efficient use of shared medical resources) are also recognized as legitimate. In this view, the physician is not obligated to give each patient any and all available treatment, but to use medical resources fairly and responsibly. Thus, while judgments, to be fair, should not be based on "social worth" criteria (or criteria such as race, class, gender, or sexual orientation), it is ethically acceptable to forgo treatments that are of marginal benefit to a patient. At least two principles are presupposed: first, that the rationale for denying treatment is reasonably related to the purposes of medicine, and second, that medical goods and services are distributed equitably, that is, in a manner that respects the fundamental equality of each patient.

A second set of ethical questions concerns the balance between the professional obligations of physicians and health care institutions and their own economic interests. The physician-patient relationship has always involved economic exchanges, but the ethical dimensions of the exchange have shifted as delivery systems have changed. Under fee-for-service medicine, providers had economic incentives to overtreat: the more tests ordered, the higher one's revenue. As long as insurers picked up the tab, both patients and physicians could remain blind to the global costs of care. Under increasingly common capitation systems, however, providers may have economic incentives to undertreat. If a provider receives fixed compensation for all patients covered by a particular plan, the less spent on each patient, the higher the provider's share. The ethical test for any payment arrangement is whether financial incentives or disincentives encourage inappropriate or substandard care.

As we have seen, assisted reproduction remains largely a fee-for-service enterprise. The high potential for profit, the open-ended character of infertility, and the importance of infertility treatment to individuals all create conditions where overtreatment, in particular the prolonged use of treatment that is unlikely to be effective, is a serious risk. In fact, the one federal regulation we have adopted regarding treatment of infertility aims at mitigating the vulnerability of infertility patients by requiring that clinics disclose success rates accurately, that is, as "take-home baby" rates.

The practice of allocating reproductive technologies according to the ability to pay raises obvious questions of fairness. If reproductive technologies are to be made available as a medical treatment, should the rich infertile have access to treatment while the poor infertile do not? It is often argued that the most basic criterion for the receipt of medical services is a disease or an impairment for which professional help is needed. If this is so, is it just to privilege those who can afford care if the disease or the impairment is the same? What are the consequences of patterns of allocation that make infertility a disease of the upper middle class? One danger is that the emphasis on high-tech interventions that follows deflects attention from the social and medical causes of infertility, some of which, such as untreated sexually transmitted diseases and undertreated endometriosis, disproportionately affect poor women and women of color. A more serious consequence, however, is that unacknowledged social worth criteria are smuggled into medical judgments. That is, inequalities of access mask social judgments about who is fit to reproduce. The demographics of assisted reproduction reflect longstanding patterns in public health, domestic and international: Where poor women are concerned, resource allocation aims at reducing fertility rather than at promoting reproductive health as it is broadly understood.

Problems of justice within assisted reproduction cannot be separated, however, from the systemic problems we currently face. It is widely agreed that the goal of expanding access to health care for the uninsured cannot be achieved by increasing health care expenditures. Although some health economists believe that market competition will bring about a cost-effective system, it is unlikely that either goal—cost-containment or securing access for the uninsured—will be realized without a reassessment of our health care priorities. No case for addressing disparities in access to procreative services, therefore, can be made without accounting for the financial impact of widely available specialized technology on an overburdened system. However, it is far from obvious, as it is often taken to be, that we should not even raise the question of equitable access to assisted reproduction when such a large number of people in the United States are without adequate access to basic medical care. The latter is a serious problem. But it is not solved by pitting one group that is, at least on the face of it, disadvantaged in the system against another. Framing the question as a zero-sum-contest between competing interests merely avoids the crucial ethical, economic, and political questions we need to face: How are costs to be contained and resources distributed efficiently in order to

satisfy human needs and desires? How do we structure our health care system
so that goods are distributed fairly and so that we are able to provide equitable
access to affordable care?[48]

Containing health care expenditures will most likely require explicit, systemic rationing. Guaranteeing equitable access will certainly require it. "Rationing" implies more than simply eliminating unwanted, excess, or "futile"
care. Systemic, explicit rationing is an agreement to deny some goods and services that are both desired and medically beneficial. It is in the context of the
moral and political inevitability of health care rationing that access to assisted
reproductive technologies must be addressed. However, developing public rationales for assigning priority in a table of health care goods is exceedingly difficult. It is no wonder that macroallocation problems are considered the most
intractable problems in medical ethics or that here in the United States we have
gone to such lengths to avoid taking up the challenge of reform. In addition to
finding reasonably objective and publicly defensible principles for denying
"low priority" care, there is the deeper problem of coming to some agreement
on health care priorities. What sort of human needs and desires ought we to be
concerned about satisfying? Exactly what does efficient and fair distribution in
health care mean? Suppose we accept the argument that a just society should
guarantee access to a decent minimum level of health care. What is a decent
minimum, given the available standard of care?

By its very nature, assisted reproduction poses some special challenges
with respect to the ethics of health care distribution. To begin with, the treatment is controversial, a point to which we will return in the next chapter. So,
while the request for access to advanced infertility services is something like
a request for kidney dialysis (that is, it is one health care claim among others),
it is also quite different. While we might ask how many end-stage renal failure
patients can be treated with dialysis given present resources, who they ought
to be or how they ought to be chosen, hardly anyone asks whether in principle
dialysis is a good thing. With reproductive technology, the means is as much a
matter of moral concern as the end.

Moreover, because it is a problem usually affecting couples rather than
individuals, infertility does not easily fit into a table of "diseases" or "impairments." As we noted earlier, the recipient of fertility services is not always infertile. In a procedure using artificial insemination with a genetic and
gestational surrogate, the woman receiving "treatment" is not infertile. In the
same way, when in vitro or embryo transfer (ET) is used to treat male factor
infertility, for example, to address low sperm motility, the site for most of the
treatment (follicle stimulation, oocyte retrieval, in vitro fertilization, and embryo transfer) is the *female* partner's body. She may exhibit no reproductive
impairment herself, except the "impairment" of having married an infertile or
subfertile man. Nor are all those who receive infertility services childless.
Since one can become infertile in a variety of ways (for example, through re-

marriage or menopause) it is possible to seek procreative services despite already having biological offspring.[49]

It has also proven difficult, as we have seen, to come to a public consensus about what kind of health care claim infertility represents. Since IVF can provide an infant but cannot reverse the condition of infertility, it is often argued that there is no social obligation to guarantee access to treatment. There is no social obligation, in other words, to address disappointments or satisfy desires. This argument has important weaknesses. Many forms of involuntary childlessness do result from pathologies of the reproductive system (e.g., malformations in sperm production, endometriosis, and missing or blocked fallopian tubes). Moreover, to distinguish between serving desires and serving needs for purposes of allocation assumes a sharp consensus on the meaning of "health-related need," that does not exist. Individuals receive hip replacements as much because they desire to regain mobility or because they are frustrated in their pursuit of pleasurable activities as because there exists an underlying pathology that can be surgically corrected. We accept repair of torn cartilage as a response to a "medical" need, whatever the motivation for having it repaired—to alleviate pain, to return to work, or to continue a daily round of golf. However, the crisis facing our health care system will require that we put the brakes on an ever-expanding concept of "need," and it will not be easy to adjudicate conflicting claims. It is difficult, however necessary, to know how to judge the importance of having children for a woman approaching her mid-30s versus the importance of maintaining physical independence for a man recently retired or the importance of waging a good fight against cancer for the patient with a poor prognosis. Oregon's efforts to arrive at consensus on a list of Medicaid priorities showed the promise of community participation in shaping health care policy, but it also illustrated the difficulty of developing objective standards for ranking the value of a medical intervention and the degree to which social location and prevailing cultural values affect understandings of quality of life.

In addition, the backdrop for asking whether access to advanced infertility services should or should not be guaranteed includes not only the reality of limited medical resources but the fact of global population pressures. Precisely because we are concerned here with *procreative* technologies, legitimate questions of justice involve the distribution of goods and services in general as well as the distribution of health care goods. Many have questioned the importance of meeting personal needs or desires or rights to bear genetically related children in a world that does not, objectively, need any more children. Some feminists have objected to a perceived inattention on the part of women who seek access to assisted reproduction to the needs of existing children in the foster care system and a disconnection between concern for "third-world" population problems and "first-world" infertility problems.[50] Thus, a further challenge for any analysis of the demands of justice with respect to assisted reproduction is the relationship between fertility as an individual value and fertility (or childbearing) as a social value. Whether or not individuals should be free, in a moral sense, to have as many children as they wish depends not only on the importance we ascribe to reproduction but also on the level of social sources available and the impact of reproductive choices on the ability of a society to meet basic needs.

As we have seen, disparities in access to infertility treatment raise questions of *micro*allocation, that is, about who ought to receive whatever goods and services are available. They also raise questions of *macro*allocation. They prompt us to account for how much we will spend on health care and how exactly we will spend it. They raise another sort of ethical question as well.

In his well-known work, *The Four Cardinal Virtues,* Josef Pieper writes: "Whoever speaks of distributive justice has to speak of exercise of power. What is under discussion is the right order in the relation between those who have power and those who are entrusted or delivered to this power."[51] Drawing on Thomas Aquinas, he argues that the demands of distributive justice pertain principally to those entrusted with the authority to distribute the goods of the community, but not exclusively; the ruled also realize distributive justice as they "are contented by a just distribution."[52]

Pieper's observation is critical for understanding what is at stake in debates over access to health care or, in this case, to a particular kind of health care. Health care, like other social goods such as food, shelter, education, and the media of communication, is necessary for the development and exercise of human capacities. Financing and dispensing health care is an exercise of social power. Of course, in assessing whether or not social power is being exercised justly under a particular system of health care distribution we need to ask what human capacities ought to be protected or promoted for the sake of dignity and the common good and how far the obligation to protect or promote them extends. But, as Pieper reminds us, it is equally important to inquire into the conditions for "right relation" between those who have power and those who are "entrusted or delivered to this power." "Right relation" can mean a variety of things in this context, as we will see. However, it means at least paying attention to the degree to which the needs of those denied some good under a certain set of arrangements are addressed and the possibilities that exist for members of a community to be "contented by a just distribution."

NOTES

1 Tamara L. Callahan, Janet E. Hall, Susan L. Ettner, Cindy L. Christiansen, Michael F. Greene, and William F. Crowley, Jr. "The Economic Impact of Multiple-Gestation Pregnancies and the Contribution of Assisted-Reproduction Techniques to Their Incidence," *New England Journal of Medicine* 331, no. 4 (July 28, 1994): 247.
2 Rick Lyman, "As Octuplets Remain in Peril, Ethical Questions are Raised," *New York Times* (December 22, 1998), A1.
3 White House Domestic Policy Council. *The President's Health Security Plan: The Complete Draft and Final Reports of the White House Domestic Policy Council* (New York: Times Books, 1993), 4.
4 Ibid., p. 34. Interestingly, in the final report of the White House Domestic Policy Council, released as "Health Security: The President's Report to the American People" on October 27, 1993, the text referring to excluded benefits reads: "Not everything is covered in the benefits package. It would be just too expensive. Examples of services that are not covered include: services that are not medically necessary or appropriate; a private room in a hospital; adult eyeglasses and contact lenses; hearing aids; cosmetic surgery." Specific references to in vitro fertilization and sex change therapy are omitted.
5 See American Society for Reproductive Medicine, "Update on Insurance Matters" [http://www.asrm.org/patients/insurance.html].
6 D'Andra Millsap, "Sex, Lies, and Health Insurance: Employer-Provided Health Insurance Coverage of Abortion and Infertility Services and the ADA," *American Journal of Law and Medicine* 23, no. 1 (1996): 59–61.
7 See, for example, *Egert v. Connecticut General Life Insurance Co.*, 900 F. 2d 1032, 1037 (7th Cir. 1990); *Ralston v. Connecticut General Life Insurance Co.*, 617 So. 2d 1379, 1381–81 (La. Ct. App. 1993). The court argued in Ralston that "Mrs. Ralston's 'sickness' is that her reproductive organs, viewed in the totality of their function, are not serving their intended pur-

pose because of a malfunction . . ." as cited in Millsap, "Sex, Lies, and Health Insurance," 57, fn. 52.

8 Milissa R. O'Rourke, "The Status of Infertility Treatments and Insurance Coverage: Some Hopes and Frustrations," *San Diego Law Review* 37 (1992): 343, 357.

9 *Ralston v. Connecticut General Life Insurance Co,* 617 So. 2d 1379, 1381–81 (La. Ct. App. 1993).

10 See *Regnier v. Industrial Commission*, 707 P. 2d 333, 336 (Ariz. Ct. App. 1985) cited in Millsap, 58, fn. 62.

11 846 F. 2d 416 (7th Cir. 1988).

12 Millsap, "Sex, Lies, and Health Insurance," 59.

13 FINRRAGE has called IVF "experimental" largely because the long-range effects on women's health of routinely used practices such as controlled ovarian hyperstimulation are unknown. That sense of "experimental" is not being disputed here. Generally speaking, that is not the sense of "experimental" at work in patterns of IVF exclusion.

14 Cost was also the reason given to lobbyists for Resolve and the American Fertility Society for exclusion of IVF from the basic benefits package in the draft Clinton plan.

15 Sharon Begley, "The Baby Myth," *Newsweek,* September 4, 1995, 38, 40. The number of IVF procedures performed increased from 3,921 in 1985 to 31,900 in 1993.

16 Ibid. Also, U.S. Congress, Office of Technology Assessment, *Infertility: Medical and Social Choices* (Washington, D.C.: U.S. Government Printing Office, 1988), chapter 8.

17 B. J. Van Voorhis, D. W. Stovall, B. D. Allen, and C. H. Syrop, "Cost-effective Treatment of the Infertile Couple," *Fertility and Sterility* 70, no. 6 (December 1988): 995–1005; C. Posacl, M. Camus, K. Osmanagaoglu, and P. Devroey, "Tubal Surgery in the Era of Assisted Reproductive Technology; Clinical Options," *Human Reproduction* 14, Supplement 1 (September, 1999): 120–36.

18 U.S. Congress, Office of Technology Assessment, *Infertility,* 148.

19 Ibid., 143.

20 As a practical matter, it is difficult to separate what is fertility related and what is not. For example, treatment for endometriosis is fertility related, although women seek treatment for reasons of general health as well. Some drugs used in assisted reproduction, such as Lupron, are routinely covered by insurance plans because they are prescribed for other purposes, such as hormonal treatment of prostate cancer.

21 Callahan et al., "The Economic Impact of Multiple-Gestation Pregnancies," 244.

22 Ibid.

23 Ibid.

24 Peter J. Neumann, Soheyla D. Gharib, and Milton C. Weinstein, "The Cost of a Successful Delivery with in Vitro Fertilization," *New England Journal of Medicine* 331, no. 4 (July 28, 1994): 239–43.

25 Ibid., 239, 240.

26 M. Griffin and W. F. Panak, "The Economic Cost of Infertility-related Services: An Examination of the Massachusetts Infertility Insurance Mandate," *Fertility and Sterility* 70, no. 1 (1998): 22–29.

27 An exception to this would be the prioritization of medical goods under the Oregon plan. The plan has been criticized for taking as its focus a specific population (Medicaid patients) and taking too little account of the views of the disabled in weighing the value of certain treatments. But the exercise was an attempt to achieve this kind of public consensus.

28 U.S. Congress, Office of Technology Assessment, *Infertility;* John A. Collins, Maria Bustillo, Robert D. Visscher, and Lynne D. Lawrence, "An Estimate of the Cost of in Vitro Fertilization Services in the United States in 1995," *Fertility and Sterility* 64 no. 3 (September 1995): 538–45.

29 S. Henshaw and M. Orr, "The Need and Unmet Need for Infertility Services in the United States, *Family Planning Perspectives* 19, no. 4 (1987): 180–83, 186.

30 At least in the population studied, Callahan et al. showed that women with twin and higher-order multiple gestation pregnancies were more likely to be older, white, and to have comprehensive health insurance (commercial insurance or HMO) than mothers of singletons. Pregnancy-related services are generally covered under Medicaid, and the 1980 Title X guidelines included the provisions of infertility services in federally funded family planning programs. However, no additional funds were allotted for this purpose. Consequently, studies show that less than 5 percent of those receiving infertility services are at poverty level or below. Henshaw and Orr, "The Need and Unmet Need for Infertility Services in the United States," 180–86; also U.S. Congress, Office of Technology Assessment, *Infertility,* chapter 8.

31 Daniel Callahan, "Cloning: The Work Not Done," *Hastings Center Report*, 27. no. 5 (September–October 1997): 18.

32 George Annas "Going Too Far?" *People,* January 18, 1999, 104.

33 Charles Dougherty, *Back to Reform: Values, Markets and the Health Care System,* (New York: Oxford University Press, 1996), 11.

34 Gene Outka, "Social Justice and Equal Access to Health Care," in *On Moral Medicine,* 2nd ed., (Grand Rapids, Mich.: William B. Eerdmans Publishing Co., 1998), 952. Under managed care arrangements, patients are often also very restricted with respect to their ability to comparison shop.

35 Peter J. Neumann, Soheyla D. Gharib, and Milton C. Weinstein, "The Cost of a Successful Delivery with in Vitro Fertilization," *The New England Journal of Medicine* 331, no. 4 (July 28, 1994): 241.

36 Z. Stern, N. Laufer, R. Levy, D. Ben-Shushan, and S. Mor-Yosef, "Cost Analysis of in Vitro Fertilization," *Israel Journal of Medical Sciences* 31, no. 8 (August 1995): 492–96.

37 Michael R. Soules, "Now That We've Painted Ourselves in a Corner," *Fertility and Sterility* 66, no. 5 (November 1996): 694. FDA regulations in the United States account in part for the higher price of new drugs, of course, but do not alone explain the persistent high price of fertility drugs like Pergonal which have been on the market for years.

38 Michael R. Soules, "Now That We've Painted Ourselves in a Corner," *Fertility and Sterility,* 66, no. 5 (November 1996): 694.

39 Ibid., 695.

40 Ibid., 693.

41 D. Frankfurter, C. B. Barrett, M. N. Alper, M. J. Berger, S. P. Oskowitz, A. S. Penzias, I. E. Thompson, and R. H. Reindollar, "Insurance Mandates for IVF Coverage Effectively Lower Multiple Births per Embryo Transfer," ASRM Annual Meeting (San Francisco, October 6, 1998).

42 Milt Freudenheim, "With A Difficult Road Ahead, HMO's are set for many more mergers," *New York Times* (January 4, 1999), C8.

43 Larry Churchill, "Market Meditopia: A Glimpse at American Health Care in 2005," *Hastings Center Report* 27, no. 1 (January–February 1997): 5.

44 Charles Dougherty, *Back to Reform*, 9–10.

45 Karen G. Gervais, Reinhard Priester, Dorothy E. Vawter, Kimberly K. Otte, and Mary M. Solberg. *Ethical Challenges in Managed Care: A Casebook* (Washington, D.C.: Georgetown University Press, 1999), 4.

46 Ibid., 5.

47 See Tom L. Beauchamp and LeRoy Walters, *Contemporary Issues in Bioethics,* 4th ed. (Belmont, Calif.: Wadsworth Publishing Co., 1994), 675–82, for an overview of problems of justice in health care.

48 Ibid., 675.

49 One study estimates that primary infertility (or "involuntary childlessness") accounts for approximately 30 percent of infertility among American couples. See M. B. Hirsch and W. D. Mosher, "Characteristics of Infertile Women in the United States and Their Use of Infertility Services," *Fertility and Sterility* 47 (1987): 618–25.

50 The United Nations Population Fund estimated in April of 1992 that the world's population would rise from 5.48 billion in mid-1992 to 10 billion in 2050, before leveling off at 11.6 billion after the year 2150. Ninety-seven percent of the increase is expected to occur in developing countries, with Africa accounting for 34 percent of the increase. Even with somewhat revised and more modest estimates, demographers warn that current rates of growth heighten the risk of future economic and ecological catastrophe. Steady or rising fertility rates in developing regions are in contrast, however, with declining rates in developed countries. Fertility rates in the

United States, for example, dropped from 2.6 births per woman in 1970 to 1.8 births per woman in 1990. See Paul Lewis, "Curb on Population Growth Needed Urgently, U.N. Says," *New York Times* (April 30, 1992), A12. First published in United Nations Department of International Economic and Social Affairs, *The World's Women 1970–1990: Trends and Statistics* (New York: United Nations Publications, 1991), 11–29.
51 Josef Pieper, *The Four Cardinal Virtues* (Notre Dame, Ind.: University of Notre Dame Press, 1966), 81 (first published 1954).
52 Ibid., 95.

CHAPTER TWO

THE ETHICS OF ASSISTED REPRODUCTION

I ask myself over and over again: Could I do this; is it sweet, the height of sisterliness, all this sharing of bodies and body parts? Or is it a transgression of some basic order, of nature itself, herself, and of the very notion of maternity?

—Anne Taylor Fleming, *Motherhood Deferred: A Woman's Journey*

Assisted reproductive technologies are ambiguous. Even when it is successful, high tech infertility treatment takes a toll on patients' lives—their emotional health, their marriages, their jobs, and, of course, their bank accounts. And even for those who welcome the therapeutic possibilities opened by IVF and its relatives [e.g., gamete intrafallopian transfer (GIFT) and zygote intrafallopian transfer (ZIFT)], assisted reproduction raises serious and persistent ethical questions.

This book is not about the ethics of assisted reproduction per se. I have not set out to offer a comprehensive analysis of the ethical problems associated with assisted reproduction or to stake positions on various interventions. Except where the very latest advances in assisted reproduction are concerned, that terrain is already well traveled, and if the growth of assisted reproduction as an industry is any indication, many people have come to terms already with their own ethical qualms about the technology. My interest is in the questions that have not yet received much attention: Where should we place assisted reproduction in a table of heath care priorities? Who should have access to treatments such as in vitro fertilization, and how should we decide? What range of services ought to be available, if in fact we think some ought to be?

But some readers will dismiss these questions as moot. We ought not be doing IVF at all, they will argue, let alone trying to decide the meaning of "fair" access. Others will take the Vatican's near blanket opposition as evidence that it is foolish to pose such questions from the perspective of Catholic social teaching. If assisted reproduction in virtually every form is incompatible with Catholic moral values, is there not something a bit disingenuous about drawing on the account of the common good rooted in that tradition, as we intend to do? Such objections can be successfully answered. As we will see, Lisa Sowle Cahill shows that it is possible to defend the use of assisted reproduction in a way that is faithful to the Catholic moral tradition's commitment to the integrity of sexuality and reproduction. However, if we are to make a case for it as a potentially valuable human or social good, we need to take seriously the moral questions posed by assisted reproduction, such as the question of its impact on our understandings of the meaning of sexuality and embodiment and our respect for the limits of power and agency.

The Ethics of Assisted Reproduction

In a broad sense, the term "assisted reproduction" refers to a wide range of biomedical/technical interventions aimed at initiating conception or managing pregnancy and parturition. Thus, it encompasses everything from genetic screening, amniocentesis, and fetal monitoring to artificial insemination and IVF and embryo transfer (ET). As I am using it here, "assisted reproduction" refers to interventions aimed at the promotion of pregnancy and includes those practices such as IVF that make use of capabilities developed in the last twenty-five years.

In general, ethical concerns about assisted reproduction can be grouped under two categories: problems related to the *means* used in assisting reproduction and problems related to the social, economic, and political context in which assisted reproduction is practiced.[1]

Questions of Means

The ability to separate the components of human reproduction and to exercise ever greater control over the processes of fertilization, embryo transfer, and gestation has been controversial since the birth of the first IVF baby in 1978. The difficulty of evaluating the moral status of the pre-embryo and embryo, which has proved so contentious in the debate over legalized abortion, emerges in this context as well. Technological reproduction has carried with it questions regarding the freezing of embryos, the ownership and disposal of non-implanted (surplus) embryos, and the possibility of research on human embryos. In addition, when multiple pregnancy results from infertility treatment, selective abortion may be recommended to guarantee the best chance of a successful gestation for the fetus or fetuses that remain.

For many people, these practices intensify qualms about the boundaries of ethically defensible intervention into fetal life or development. The Vatican's "Instruction on Respect for Human Life in Its Origin and on the Dignity of Procreation (*Donum Vitae*)," published by the Congregation for the Doctrine of the Faith in 1987 in order to answer questions for Roman Catholics and Roman Catholic institutions concerning the use of reproductive technology, captures the worry that assisted reproduction involves an illicit tampering with the very "stuff" of human existence:

> *[The process that consists of] IVF and ET is brought about outside the bodies of the couple through actions of third parties whose competence and technical activity determine the success of the procedure. Such fertilization entrusts the life and identity of the embryo to the power of doctors and biologists and establishes the domination of technology over the origin and destiny of the human person.*[2]

The character of IVF as a "gateway" to the therapeutic and experimental manipulation of human embryos raises deep concerns about the potential for abuse or exploitation of potential human life. Recent controversy over embryo stem cell research illustrates both the depth of anxieties over the potential of such practices to erode respect for human life and the extent of existing disagreement over the nature of the early embryo. Primordial stem cells can serve as an invaluable source for human tissue. However, the two principal sources of cells are aborted fetuses and spare embryos from fertility treatment (which must be destroyed in the research process). Those who hold a developmental view of the moral status of the pre-embryo see little problem, in principle, with using spare embryos for stem cell research and most would allow the use of tissue obtained through elective abortion. Before the embryo is individualized, it need not command the full protection paid to human subjects. The only ethical questions, therefore, concern the conduct of the research. But for those who hold that there exists a full human person, in the moral sense, from the moment of conception, stem cell research is inherently unethical. In the statement to the *New York Times*, theologian Nigel Cameron of Trinity International University in northern Illinois expressed this position well: "Here is one of us [the embryo], however primitive, and the question is whether members of the human species should be treated as other than ends in themselves."[3]

Some critics of technological reproduction worry about the broader and subtler effects of increased human mastery over nascent life. To what extent, they wonder, does technological reproduction in itself reflect dangerous scientific hubris? What happens to human creatureliness when technological skill replaces nature or God as the acknowledged "author" of life? Is the "human" aspect of reproduction lost when conception is accomplished in the laboratory rather than in the act of sexual intercourse? As Gilbert Meilaender argues in *Body, Soul and Bioethics*, what is at stake in resistance to assisted reproduction from this point of view is our very ability to understand what is human in the act of bringing forth offspring:

[W]hen we dismember procreation into its several parts and combine them in new and different ways, we simply enact a new myth of creation in which human beings are created with two separate faculties—one manifesting the deepening unity of the partners through sexual relations, the other giving rise to children through a "cool, deliberate act of man's rational will." . . . We should not assume . . . that those who "procreate" and those who—having severed procreation into its parts—"reproduce" are doing the same thing.[4]

Anxieties generated by the power to manipulate human reproduction—to "handle" the human embryo—are part of the deeper societal anxieties over control which accompany the acquisition of new and life-altering knowledge. Appreciation for human mastery is often sobered by the memory of our human capacities for evil. Some observers warn that reproductive technologies unleash abilities that cannot be contained or that expand the dangerous temptations of knowledge and power. They fear that reproductive technologies may be impossible to confine to therapeutic use, that technology developed to treat clinical infertility will be used to facilitate mass governmental breeding, or to create fetuses for experimentation, or to institutionalize commercial reproduction for "convenience." They worry also that procedures for artificial reproduction, which can incorporate genetic engineering, will be employed intentionally for eugenic purposes. Frequently cited possibilities for abuse range from the sinister (e.g., the use of artificial reproduction and genetic engineering technology to produce a "super race") to the "unreflectively" eugenic (that is, the promotion of a standard of reproductive excellence that makes health, intelligence, race, or gender criteria for the acceptability of offspring).

How to protect reproductive agency against the encroachment of technical expertise has been an important question for feminists in the evaluation of assisted reproduction. Although feminists are sharply divided in their appraisal of the new reproductive technologies, they are agreed on this much: History demonstrates that women's sexual, procreative, and nurturing capacities have regularly been manipulated, exploited, and appropriated to accommodate societal interests.[5] Thus, advances which increase the range of human control over the processes of reproduction are never neutral. Although, as I mentioned earlier, some feminists have seen the ability to re-create maternity technologically as a powerful moment in women's biological and social liberation, in general feminists have been wary of the promises of assisted reproduction to serve or empower women. As Margaret Farley cautions, removing conception from the body has serious implications for women's sense of embodiment:

Women's previous experience with reproductive technology suggests that women's own agency is likely to be submerged in the network of

> *multiple experts needed to achieve in vitro fertilization. Far from this ac-*
> *complishing liberation for women from childbearing responsibilities, it*
> *can entail "further alienation of our life processes."*[6]

For most feminists, the removal of reproduction from women's bodies has serious political implications as well. Under virtually universal conditions of
gender inequality, medically assisted reproduction risks becoming a means
through which women lose their unique maternal power, their place as "bear-
ers of the gift of life." What begins as a promise to increase reproductive
agency may end instead with women realizing that they have simply given it
over more completely to men—as scientists and technicians, as well as biological fathers. The risk of the technological revolution, cautions Gina Corea,
is that women will become finally redundant. It is not impossible to imagine
that our daughters could someday come to think of reproduction as "a complicated intellectual and technical feat performed by teams of highly skilled
men who use, as raw material for their achievements, the body parts of a variety of interchangeable females."[7]

   The ability to separate the components of reproduction gives rise not
only to concerns about the proper treatment of the embryo and the legitimate
scope of reproductive intervention, but also to questions about the nature of the
family and the social function of procreation. Recognition that a newborn
could begin life with five parents (egg donor, sperm donor, gestational mother,
and two rearing parents), each of whose legal and moral relationship to the
child is not a priori obvious, calls long-held assumptions about family and parenting into question. From one point of view, greater flexibility in defining a
"family" is welcome. Challenges to the norm of the biological or nuclear family are not only more reflective of contemporary social realities, but aid in
breaking down ideologies that have contributed to the oppression of women
and the abuse of children. On the other hand, concerns are voiced that technological reproduction threatens to blur fundamental human bonds. It thereby
poses potentially serious identity problems for the offspring of such arrangements, and it disrupts the traditional notion of parentage (making it a matter of
contract to nurture more than one of nature). Since much of the public debate
over the technology has been generated by disputes over rights to offspring,
much legal energy thus far has been directed toward the definition of roles and
responsibilities under reproductive contracts.

   It is not only the complexities of identity, kinship, maternity, and paternity that are at issue in current responses to reproductive technology, but also
the nature of heterosexual marriage and its function as a reproductive unit.
Reproductive technology allows for procreation by single individuals without
sexual intercourse, by lesbian and gay couples, and potentially by women
without male involvement. It even offers possibilities for interspecies gestation. Heterosexual marriage as the culturally sanctioned context for repro-

duction (at least in the West) is therefore challenged and potentially undermined. Once again, those who see heterosexual marriage as a breeding ground for sexual inequality take the erosion of cultural ideals of the family as a positive step; but for those who view the nuclear family as the primary social unit, the core interpersonal arena, where communal values are preserved and passed on, the real or symbolic disruption of the family is a societal loss of enormous proportions.

Assisted reproduction also challenges the symbolic unity of marriage, sexual intercourse, and procreation. In the Roman Catholic tradition, as in other religious traditions, children are viewed as the physical manifestation of a married couple's deep and enduring love. Under this description, the child serves as a witness to the "one-flesh unity" of the parents and to the fruitfulness of their committed love.[8] The concern that techniques such as artificial insemination and in vitro fertilization destroy the mutually conditioning relationship between marital love and parenthood by separating procreation from sexual intercourse is at least as central to the Vatican's resistance to assisted reproduction as concerns about the treatment of embryos. *Donum Vitae* argues:

> *[F]rom the moral point of view, procreation is deprived of its proper perfection when it is not desired as the fruit of the conjugal act, that is to say, of the specific act of the spouses' union. . . . The moral relevance of the link between the meanings of the conjugal act and between the goods of marriage, as well as the unity of the human being and the dignity of his origin, demand that the procreation of a human person be brought about as the fruit of a conjugal act specific to the love between spouses.[9]*

Underlying the "Instruction's" insistence on the integrity of procreation within "the marital embrace" is a certain interpretation of human dignity as well as a certain understanding of the meaning of sexuality. In a move that even many of those sympathetic to its conclusions found problematic, *Donum Vitae* asserted the right of the child to be "the fruit of a specific act of the conjugal love of its parents."[10] The invocation of rights language in that context is by most accounts unfortunate, but what it intends to express is the danger many others have also noted of objectifying children who come about through "acts of will" and the exercise of the experts' skills.

> *In his unique and irrepeatable origin, the child must be respected and recognized as equal in personal dignity to those who give him life. . . . He cannot be desired or conceived as the product of an intervention of medical or biological techniques; that would be equivalent to reducing him to an object of scientific technology.[11]*

When assisted reproduction involves the use of donors to provide gametes or gestational services, it introduces additional parties into the reproductive relationship. The potential for confusion in familial roles and loss of genetic heritage leads many people to reject donor-assisted reproduction, even if they find nothing objectionable in the idea of assisted reproduction. The concern is that such practices not only threaten the symbolic integrity of marriage, but also create a potentially serious imbalance in the parenting relationship (since often in these arrangements only one rearing parent is biologically related to the offspring). Given that the importance of biological parentage is one of the primary values driving the development and application of this technology, this is a more significant and complex consideration than it may appear. The question is: Will artificial reproduction undermine the co-parental relationship even while it makes an individual case of genetic parenting possible at all?

The growing use of donors in assisted reproduction prompts ethical questions that relate both to means and context. While the practice of maintaining secrecy regarding an adoptive child's origins is gradually giving way to the popularity of "open" adoption, secrecy remains the norm in donor-assisted reproduction. Concerned for the rights of offspring to have access to their genetic heritage, lawmakers in some countries have outlawed donor methods and others require that genetic information be provided on request to offspring conceived through gamete donation. But the "hands-off" regulatory approach we have taken toward assisted reproduction as well as the tendency in the United States to privilege the interests of would-be parents over all other interests has meant that little attention has been paid to and little legal protection offered for the rights of offspring in donor-assisted reproduction. Whether the use of donor gametes is revealed is a matter of parental choice. Some critics charge that important questions of informed consent are overlooked: The freedom to have control over one's own genetic information is a priori violated under a veil of deception about the circumstances of one's birth.[12] But the deeper worry for many people is that we are adopting and institutionalizing practices that may be harmful to children (or may not) before we have the experience and wisdom to know—before, for example, we have heard from those who have been born from donated eggs or sperm. Moreover, we are introducing new forms of economic collaboration into reproduction in a culture that may not have the moral resources to manage them.

Questions of Context

In addition to the questions of distributive justice that we have already noted, various ethical issues arise from the fact that an initiating couple may purchase gametes or pay a fee for gestational services.[13] One has to do with the commercialization of reproduction per se; that is, whether a gamete or a period of gestation is the kind of thing that ought to be purchased or sold. Should the generation of human life be a subject of market relations at all? It is clear from the previous chapter that the problem of market relations does not just arise in donor-assisted forms of reproduction. However, the use of donors, in particular the increasing use of female egg donors, makes explicit the contours of new economic relationships in a way that many people find troubling. A recent advertisement placed in Ivy League college newspapers offered $50,000 for a young, tall egg donor with high SAT scores. The furor over the ad was reminiscent of the "Baby M" debate, which brought the issue of commercial surrogacy into the public spotlight. "Baby M" was born through a gestational surrogate who resisted relinquishing the child after birth. The contracting couple argued that they had entered into a good faith contract with the surrogate who had been justly paid for the service she performed. But, as people wondered in that case, when do we cross the line, from "reasonable compensation" to "baby selling," from "gamete donation" to the exchange of a "reproductive product?"

At what point, people also wondered, does commercialized assisted reproduction promote the exploitation of persons? What amount of money would fairly repay a donor for her time, inconvenience, and willingness to assume long- and short-term health risks, known and unknown, without providing an inappropriate incentive? How like or unlike organ donation is egg or sperm donation? Concerns that infertile couples are vulnerable before the professional interests of those who develop and market reproductive technologies are intensified with the growth in agencies that broker third-party arrangements. Infertile patients who need or desire to enter into donor relationships have little legal protection against being exploited by brokers. Donors are also potentially at risk, both directly and indirectly. At least some critics of third-party assisted reproduction argue that there is no just compensation for the physical and emotional risks women undertake in donating eggs or providing gestational services. Even for those who believe just compensation can be determined, the fact that egg donors are usually women in their early twenties and often persons whose own economic situation would not allow them to use the technology for their own interests raises the possibility that donors may not be wholly free and full partners to the contract.

Whether donors or infertile patients themselves have genuine freedom to choose has been long a point of contention in the assessment of reproductive technologies. The manipulation of success rates by clinics and the experimental character of the clinical development of assisted reproduction have been raised as one sort of informed consent problem. To what extent are patients contemplating IVF given accurate information concerning the probability of actually delivering a child? If they are older women, as many are, are they aware of the sharp decline in the effectiveness of IVF for women over 40? Even with the passage of the Fertility Clinic Success Rate and Certification Act, which requires clinics to publish take-home baby rates, patients must rely in large part on good faith in making treatment decisions. Compliance is voluntary and many clinics do not participate in the survey. Moreover, because most of what is known about reproductive technology is learned in "on the job" clinical experimentation, some of the risks to patients, offspring, and donors posed by the use of fertility drugs or new techniques in fertilization are unknown even to the experts. Thus, "full disclosure" may only mean "what we know today."

Even more interesting questions of informed consent have been raised by feminists skeptical about the possibilities for a free choice for motherhood in a sexist society. The pressure to fulfill the socially required role of parent creates conditions under which, feminists fear, choosing to remain childless is not a viable alternative, particularly for women. The development of medical "options" generates new burdens, with the introduction of egg donation as a case in point. Now, some worry, not even menopause "frees" women from the pressure to mother, not even the lack of eggs provides a limit condition to what one might be asked to endure for the sake of conception.

As the deep disagreements over the introduction of commercial surrogacy best illustrate, feminists have been divided over how to judge the "freedom" or "right" to exchange reproductive services in the market. Most agree that the donor relationship in commercial assisted reproduction need not be exploitative, and some, like Lori Andrews, have argued that having the right to serve as gamete donors, as men long have had, is an important step in securing procreative equality for women.[14] But many worry that donor relationships may be, if not necessarily exploitative, inherently *oppressive*. In the typical case of commercial surrogacy, for example, a white upper or upper-middle-class woman hires a genetic and/or gestational surrogate, who is a woman of lesser means, to perform a service which, in western culture, is not valued very highly (even if the "product" is valued highly). Reproductive service (such as ovum or gestational donation) is tied, at this point in history, to the other services women perform, such as housework and childcare. While this kind of reproductive service could come to occupy a higher status in a society, which has come to value all domestic services differently, there is little reason to suppose that commercializing it or institutionalizing it will change the way we think about it. Feminists argue that until the care of children and of the home is a shared task (and one not assigned by gender), it is doubtful that many women in surrogacy arrangements will be doing anything through reproductive service other than they always have done—bear children at great risk and relatively low compensation to meet others' interests in the finished product. Insofar as commercial surrogacy as an institution depends upon social conditions that guarantee the existence of women who are willing to do this, important questions of class privilege arise.

The potential for new forms of distorted relationships between "reproductively partnered strangers" underscores the importance of assessing assisted reproduction both as socially constructed and as an agent of social construction.

Concerns are raised, therefore, about the practice of assisted reproduction under a given set of social, economic, and political conditions—what incentives or disincentives will motivate choices concerning the technology, which values and rules will govern access and the disposition of gametes and human embryos, and how the experience of reproduction will be shaped as alternate ways of reproducing are introduced. The impact of assisted reproductive technologies on available methods for addressing infertility is also a concern. We have already noted the potential for developments in reproductive technology to medicalize infertility, making a multidimensional biological, social, political, and economic problem into a merely medical problem, and shifting infertility from a challenge for reproductive health generally to a problem of the "visible" infertile. An additional danger is the potential for assisted reproduction to devalue or destabilize the institution of adoption. At least some observers fear that the drive toward genetic connection that underlies motivations for assisted reproduction will undermine other forms of familial connection to children. In an ironic twist, technologies with the potential to redefine entirely our understanding of "parenthood" as a biological event could simply reaffirm the most narrow, proprietary interests in "children of my own."

This review of the ethical and theological questions raised by assisted reproduction is hardly exhaustive. It is sufficient, however, to give a sense of some of the serious concerns that need to be acknowledged in a defense of assisted reproductive technology as a response to infertility, especially a defense with both feminist and Catholic commitments. But what exactly should we make of such concerns? Can we give a principled account of assisted reproduction that supports the choice to seek a remedy in reproductive technology, perhaps even sees reproductive technology as a good in some cases?

The Case for Assisted Reproduction

In several commentaries on *Donum Vitae*, Lisa Sowle Cahill offers a justification of at least some uses of assisted reproduction that honors the moral and theological commitments that are central to a Christian or Catholic analysis.[15] As a feminist, she is sensitive as well to concerns about the impact of reproductive technologies on efforts to create a climate of equal respect and equal social power for women and men. Cahill illustrates how it is possible to affirm the value of reproductive technologies for individuals while approaching their use with appropriate caution.

At the heart of her position is a nuanced appreciation for the integrity of sexuality, marriage, and parenthood in the Catholic natural law tradition:

Parent-childhood is an embodied as well as freely chosen relationship, and it is best carried out as an extension of the mutual

spouse-parental relationship (also embodied as well as freely em-
braced) with which procreative sexual intercourse ideally connects it.
The physical or embodied aspects of marriage and parenthood are
not as important morally as those which are psychospiritual and
social. . . . However, it is crucial to recognize the unity of both aspects
of the person and of morality by giving even the subsidiary dimension
(the physical) some significant weight and role in decisions about
reproductive technologies.[16]

Cahill argues that in a Christian perspective on reproductive technologies, it is important to "appreciate the human and moral importance of biological kinship, without either absolutizing it or making its level of importance to social parenthood totally dependent on individual choice."[17] Honoring parenthood as a biological extension of marriage need not rule out assisted reproduction. *Donum Vitae's* opposition to IVF and artificial insemination even in cases where a couple's own gametes will be used is based, in her view, on a distorted understanding of the unity of sex, love, and procreation, one that ties this unity to "specific sexual *acts* rather than to the marital *relationship"*[18] To argue that procreation must take place as a direct consequence of a sexual act falsely absolutizes the relation of sexual intimacy, procreation, and parenthood. Married couples realize sexual and reproductive partnership not only in the discrete moments of conjugal relationship but throughout the course of a marriage. Even in cases where conception takes place outside of a sexual act, as in IVF, it is possible for a couple to realize the goods of marriage as defined by the tradition, that is sexual intimacy, fidelity, and openness to the gift of new life. These are goods experienced and honored, not just or even principally in their sexual relationship, but in the totality of their life together. Indeed, given the negative effect infertility can have on marital intimacy, it is possible to see assisted reproduction as a valuable way to serve those goods in some cases, enabling a couple to realize reproductive partnership while freeing sexual intimacy from the often deadening frustration of unrealized expectation.

Arguing that "the physical or embodied aspects of marriage and parenthood are not as important morally as those which are psychospiritual and social" allows Cahill to justify recourse to assisted reproduction where it is necessary in order for the infertile couple to realize reproduction. However, while the union of sexuality, reproduction, and parenthood need not be realized in an absolute sense, it remains a fundamental value in a Christian treatment of marriage. The union of sexual intimacy, procreation, and parenthood acts as a kind of boundary for thinking about choices with respect to reproduction. Procreation is a shared biological endeavor *growing out of an exclusive sexual and marital relationship*. The most obvious consequence of emphasizing the importance of the link between reproductive partnership and marital exclusivity is a critique of donor-assisted methods of reproduction.

"These methods," argues Cahill, are "premised on a preconceived intention of the donor to sever the activity of procreation from the personal relation of parenthood (vis-à-vis both the offspring and the procreative partner). . . . Third-party methods of obtaining ova or sperm intrude a third *person* on the marriage, even if he or she is supposedly affectively uninvolved and is recognized only as a biological contributor."[19]

Even if homologous methods of IVF and artificial insemination (AI) are supported in Cahill's reading of the Catholic natural law tradition, important questions remain with regard to the uses of technology in reproduction. The development of commercial markets in eggs or sperm is only the most overt illustration of the hegemony of market values in social discourse about reproduction. Privileging choice above all other considerations, and emphasizing achievement of ends over reflection on means, current discussions of reproductive practices and policies too often reflect an impoverished account of reproduction in which both its biological and social dimensions are undermined. Even the "easy" case of homologous IVF, therefore, presses commonly neglected questions for Cahill: How do we understand what we are doing not only as a choice but also as a realization of the goods of biological and social parenthood? What are the social repercussions of our choices? Thus, Cahill also incorporates concern for the controversial extensions of assisted reproduction—such as post-menopausal pregnancies, genetic engineering for purposes of enhancing human traits, and sex preselection—into an overall appreciation of the value of assisted reproduction in the promotion of genetic parenthood.

The impact of assisted reproduction on the status of women is an important social repercussion of individual choices to use reproductive technology. Although Cahill is sympathetic to the importance of pregnancy and childbearing to women, she is critical of the role of technological reproduction in reinforcing a view of female sexuality that reduces women to their reproductive capacities and that leads women and men to see "the sexual and reproductive services of women as men's natural right and due."[20] The remedy does not lie in banning reproductive technologies, as it does for some feminists. It lies here again in questioning a liberal philosophy and politics of choice that ignores the "construction of desperation," the subtle and coercive social, economic, and cultural forces that constrain possibilities for overcoming infertility.

The strength of Cahill's position is in the delicate balance she is able to strike between, on the one hand, giving the biological or genetic dimensions of human reproduction an absolute moral status and, on the other, treating biological and genetic connections as wholly dispensable. This permits her to acknowledge the human affective importance of conception, pregnancy, and childbirth, to honor the obligation and the desire to bring forth children who are "flesh of our flesh," without treating biological reproduction as a value that should be pursued at all costs. By arguing that the physical or embodied aspects of marriage and parenthood are important, but not as important morally as those which are psychospiritual and social, she opens the window to noncoital reproduction, while maintaining the status of adoption as a morally commendable alternative to assisted reproduction. In addition, it becomes possible to see, at least broadly, the boundaries on social obligations to promote biological parenting. Privileging the psychospiritual and social dimensions of parenthood places social responsibilities for the care of children above obligations to facilitate the "acquisition" of children. At the same time, the desire for biological and genetic reproduction can be acknowledged as "natural" or even as a kind of "given." It is not necessary to oppose all uses of technology in reproduction. What is important is resisting those practices, such as institutionalized gamete donation, that either undermine or ignore the interconnection of love, sex, and procreation.

Not everyone will accept Cahill's delicate balance. Those who argue that fertilization outside the body necessarily violates the moral conditions for reproduction (who hold, in other words, that the unity of sex, love, and procreation must be realized in each *act* rather than within the marriage as a whole) will reject Cahill's defense even of homologous IVF. Likewise, those feminists who believe that genuine control of reproduction for women will come only when women entirely reject medical intervention into reproduction are likely to think that Cahill is not suspicious enough of the interplay of power, gender, and economics in reproductive medicine. At least some readers of the Catholic natural law tradition will disagree that the ideal or norm for parenthood is found in the intrinsic connections of biological and social parenthood. Paul Lauritzen, for example, has argued that the core of responsible parenthood is "the commitment to, and the activities of, caring for a child in a way that promotes human flourishing."[21] To create a child with the intention of severing the genetic and social bonds does not, therefore, as Cahill suggests, threaten the "core of parenthood [or] the stringency of parental obligations."[22] It is the interpersonal bonds that define the moral relations. Others have argued that Christian ideals of parenthood have been overidentified with the Western nuclear and patriarchal family to the disadvantage of both women and children and the denigration of other forms of family association.[23]

In my view, Cahill is correct in treating the biological or genetic dimension of reproduction as subsidiary yet morally important. But Lauritzen's objection is fair. If we want to say that the unity of sex, love, and procreation is properly realized not in each act but in the whole of a marriage, and that the biological dimensions of parenthood are secondary to its psychospiritual and social dimensions, why give the parents' shared genetic relation such weight in the assessment of donor-assisted reproduction? Lauritzen may be correct that it is difficult to demonstrate empirically the risks to the care of children that Cahill and others fear in the institutionalization of third-party arrangements. It may be true, as well, that this position gives the genetic contributions of spouses too much importance in defining the embodied dimension of reproduction. As Lauritzen observes, "caring for children—however, they are conceived—is no mere assertion of the will, but is a bodily affair from start to finish."[24] Moreover, some newer methods of assisted reproduction threaten to blur almost hopelessly the boundaries between the "genetic" and the "biological" in reproduction. For example, the recipient of a donated egg does not embody genetic partnership with her spouse, but in the activity of gestation, does embody biological partnership. She brings forth a child who, while not her genetic progeny, is nonetheless the "flesh of her flesh."[25]

Still, Cahill's sketch of the boundaries captures a set of relations that are central to the meaning of reproductive partnership for the Catholic tradition. Procreation is, as we have said, a shared biological endeavor, *growing out of an exclusive sexual and marital relationship*. At stake in third-party arrangements is not only our experience and understanding of procreation, but also our experience and understanding of Christian marriage and the normative relationships between procreation and marriage. The acknowledgment that children have been and can be well cared for by persons with no genetic connection to them does not answer the question of what values we want to protect in the policies and practices we promote concerning marriage and reproduction. If, as Cahill suggests, one of the things we mean by marriage is "reproductive exclusivity," third-party arrangements have implications as much for the conceptual or symbolic foundations of marriage that we seek to protect as for the conditions we think are important for promoting the welfare of children.

In the same way, the difficulty in gathering empirical data on donor-assisted reproduction's impact on the well-being of children may temper straightforward "slippery-slope" arguments, but concerns about the impact of gamete donation on attitudes toward children and childbearing run deeper even than questions of harm to individual children. As Thomas Murray points out: "Unreflective ideological commitments can and do lead us astray, away from what we genuinely and deeply value. The attitudes and institutions that provide the absolutely necessary cultural support for what we value can be eroded, so gradually that we scarcely notice."[26] The risk in reinterpreting reproduction so that we accept the intentional, a priori severing of genetic and social parenting or institutionalize the practice of "checking one's reproductive responsibilities at the door" is that we thereby adopt practices that will erode the very attitudes and institutions that provide the support for what we value in parental-child relationships. If, as Cahill rightly argues, what we value in the unity of sex, love, and procreation in Christian tradition is the formation and expression of loving and enduring bonds, the question for donor-assisted reproduction is not really whether it possible for such bonds to form between parents and children conceived through egg or sperm donation—it is obvious that they can. The question is whether we are adopting forms of or symbolic understandings of reproduction that undermine our personal and social capacities to appreciate and embody these core reproductive and marital values.

Cahill's account of the intrinsic and normative connections between sex, love, and procreation is drawn from a specific religious tradition. As such, these connections will not be self-evident to everyone, even if our cultural languages and practices concerning marriage and reproduction show points of convergence. I agree with Cahill that a commitment to natural law moral reasoning implies an obligation to argue on grounds that are publicly intelligible, at least when public policy is to be decided. However, it is not necessary at this point to show how appeals to this religiously based account of the relation among sex, love, and procreation can be made accessible to those outside of this religious tradition. It is not clear that one would even need to appeal to normative boundaries within reproduction to find grounds for consensus on the moral problems associated with donor-assisted reproduction. Many people share Cahill's concerns about the commercialization of reproduction through gamete donation programs, for example, and many feminists are skeptical about claims that donor-assisted reproduction serves women's interests. In any case, our task is only to show that a choice to seek the help of assisted reproduction can be defended within the Catholic tradition.

What about Adoption?

It is often argued that there is something incongruous about expending social resources to create new babies when so many children (inside and outside of the United States) are not taken care of well enough. No one should have recourse to artificial reproduction, the argument goes, until all of the adoptable children in the United States are taken in—until all of the more than 400,000 children currently in foster care who need permanent homes are received into them. It does not make sense to be ambitiously fighting infertility at the same time as urban hospitals are spending over $34 million dollars a year boarding newborns who have no place to go. Or, along similar lines, it is argued that short-term social energies at least ought to be directed toward addressing the nation's scandalously high infant mortality rate, toward providing accessible pre-natal care and immunization for preventable childhood diseases. Pronatal concern should be with the 2,685 babies born into poverty in the United States every day or with the infants in sub-Saharan Africa who are dying in greater numbers than anywhere else in the world, rather than with creating new babies, some of whom will need (given the problem of multiple births) significant social resources.

These are important objections that need to be addressed. The argument that the needs of existing children place a higher moral claim on social resources than the loss of the opportunity for biological reproduction is in many

ways a compelling one, especially in light of the commitment we have made
to place assisted reproduction in the context of a common good ethic. It underscores the important and often overlooked distinction between the possession of children and the care of children, between reproductive or family
policy that is oriented toward the interests of certain adults, and policy that is
oriented toward the needs of vulnerable persons, particularly of children.
Whatever good reasons may be offered for developing reproductive technologies, the case cannot stand on a romantic or disingenuous proclamation of this
society's special affection for its young. Neither can a case for a right to assisted reproduction be advanced without attention to alternative ways of creating a family, such as adoption, and the implications of reproductive
technologies for the construction of choices concerning those alternatives.

The stark realities evoked also call attention to the larger questions of social priorities within which the particular ethical questions that attend reproductive technology must be set. They prompt reflection about equity in the
distribution of goods and in access to opportunity, about economics and
human needs, and given the demographics of urban poverty in this country,
about the role of racism in the construction of social tragedy. They point as
well to questions that need to be raised about the directions in health care policy; our high infant mortality rate is a reminder, among other things, of the
failure of the system to make effective prenatal care available.

Adoption, especially of hard to place children, can be a morally commendable response to the problems facing endangered children in our country
and our world today. Adoption can also be a healing and wonderful way to resolve the crisis of involuntary childlessness. To open one's home to a child to
whom you are not genetically related, to embrace that child as your own with
all the uncertainties that can accompany adoption, is to realize in a profound
way the ideal of the Christian family of which Cahill speaks in her most recent
book; not the nuclear family focused inward on the welfare of its own members, but the socially transformative family that seeks to make the Christian
moral ideal of love of neighbor part of the common good."[27]

It is a mistake, however, to treat assisted reproduction and adoption as
either-or answers to infertility or to assume that adoption is the obvious and
unambiguous solution to the problem of infertility. The argument that there are
too many children in the world in need of parents, or simply too many people
in the world already, to justify providing access to reproductive technologies
has considerable rhetorical power but some serious weaknesses. One problem
is that the call to adoption is almost always applied selectively. A case can be
made that all Christian couples, all Christian families have obligations to take
the needs of abandoned, neglected, or endangered children into account in
making procreative decisions. This follows, not only from the implications of
calling family life to a socially transformative neighbor-love, but from something we will develop further in the chapters to come: the obligation to assess

the social consequences of choices, especially for the most vulnerable, incumbent on all procreative decisions considered from the perspective of the common good.[28] However, as a practical matter, it is only infertile persons who are expected to assume such a duty. Fertile persons can reproduce at will, and they are not expected to match their procreative desires with the needs of the nation or of the world.

There are, of course, relevant differences between natural and assisted reproduction. Because assisted reproduction requires medical resources, it is an enterprise to which, from the outset, the questions of distributive justice legitimately apply. As we already noted, the liberty to reproduce is simply more complex when it can only be accomplished by employing potentially valuable and limited medical goods in the same way that the "liberty to breathe" is when it involves the need for a respirator. Thus, we have to acknowledge that different questions can be asked of artificial reproduction.

But the relevant differences between natural and assisted reproduction also point to an important problem with the selective call to adoption. Because they can only reproduce with medical assistance, infertile individuals are vulnerable in ways that might not make them automatically and obviously the best candidates for parenting through adoption. Many infertile individuals and couples come to see adoption as the most fitting way of resolving infertility. They get there, however, only by facing the loss of the experience of genetic parenting squarely and working through it to a different way of thinking about themselves, their family, and their future. To make a blanket assumption that infertility should be solved by adoption neglects the individual nature of the process of healing and the fact that not all infertile people will come to the place where they are able to positively embrace adoption. The many adoptable children who have special needs of some kind are not necessarily going to be well taken care of by someone for whom such an adoption is not really a positive and free choice. As Mary Midgley and Judith Hughes observed, human love is not the kind of thing which, like a liquid, can be made to flow in one direction simply by being prevented from flowing in another.[29] The kind of love that children need, in particular children with special problems, can be cultivated but it cannot be required. In this sense, one could argue for a greater obligation to adopt on the part of the fertile who would not, in principle, begin with the same vulnerabilities.

There are deeper problems with linking access to reproductive technologies to national or international child welfare. It is both false and dangerous to draw a simple correlation, as is frequently done, between not providing access to reproductive technologies and improving the situation of the many children in need. It is true that adoption provides families for children without them and children for parents without them. However, the relationship between the care of at-risk children and choices to adopt is not a simple one-to-one equation. For one thing, the infertile who turn to adoption are often interested, for both good and bad reasons, in adopting healthy, white infants. As such, adoption by the infertile addresses just one part of the problem of parentless children.[30]

More important, the social problems that account for the numbers of at-risk children in our country or our world are not simply problems of children without parents. They are problems generated by, among other things, race and class stratification, by economic systems that are not designed to serve the needs of children or the health of families, and by cultural ideologies of the family which privatize the obligations of child nurture. More people choosing the option of adopting at-risk children would be valuable in attending to the needs of individual children. But to suggest that the problems of poverty, malnutrition, marital breakdown, substance abuse—and internationally, war, disease, migration, "overpopulation"—that account for parentless children can be solved by denying access to reproductive technology grossly oversimplifies reality. This position denies the basic fact that, as Germaine Greer put it so well, "fewer people will not necessarily mean more to go round, because we are not yet committed to making it go round in the first place."[31] We are not committed to distributing resources equitably, organizing our economic and political systems to serve human needs, or caring for children as a national priority. Medically assisted reproduction has implications for addressing the social problems that endanger so many children. It involves important choices about resources and how they will be spent. Moreover, practices that give a high priority to genetic parentage contribute to a tendency to make the care of children a private rather than public or collective concern. However, limiting access to reproductive technology does not attend to these deeper issues, and, in fact, obscures them.

Two conclusions can be drawn concerning the relation of adoption to arguments for access to medically assisted reproduction in a Christian ethic. First, it is reasonable to argue that Christian families have a prima facie duty of hospitality to those most in need in their community in proportion to their financial, emotional, and physical abilities.[32] Infertile couples may, by virtue of their infertility, have a special opportunity to reach out to a child in need. Steps can and should be taken to encourage adoption, such as support for an adoption tax credit and for employer-sponsored adoption benefit programs. However, a distinction must be made between a responsibility to take into account the social costs of a reproductive decision and/or to consider adoption as means of building a family, and a responsibility not to pursue medically assisted reproduction. The latter way of construing the moral duty involved neglects the possibility of differential capacities for hospitality and undermines the complexity of the relationship between adoptable children and choices about social investments.

Second, cultivating the ability to take into account the social implications of reproductive choices or to see the connections between one's pursuit of a child of one's own and the vulnerability of children at the margins, is an important task for faith communities. The willingness to embrace adoption, especially in the midst of coping with infertility, or the power to decide against the pursuit of assisted reproduction out of a commitment to social justice, does not grow in a vacuum. As we will see in the next chapter, infertility presents a profound crisis of the self. It arises at the juncture between one's own hopes and dreams for the future and socially constructed and imposed roles and expectations. It is a crisis that can be resolved in a variety of ways, medical and nonmedical. It can be resolved without ever becoming a parent or without ever having a child. Overcoming the crisis, however, is a matter of transcending the losses posed by infertility, refashioning an understanding of the self, and rethinking one's connection to the community. There are resources for transcendence in the Christian tradition, in the call to neighbor-love of which Cahill speaks, for example, or in the image of the body of Christ, in which we are joined by spiritual rather than biological ties. These resources need to be marshaled in a compassionate and holistic response to infertility, one that not only offers alternatives to the medical pursuit of parenthood, but also asks what would make it possible for individuals and couples to pursue those alternatives.

Reproduction and the Common Good

At least two themes or values emerge in this cautious defense of assisted reproduction from the standpoint of Catholic or Christian ethics. One is the moral significance of *embodiment*. We see here that any analysis of reproduction or reproductive technologies will be impoverished insofar as it treats the body as simply the "raw material for choice," or as a neutral site for scientific experimentation. The point of departure for a moral tradition that takes its bearings from a Thomistic account of human flourishing, as does the Catholic tradition, is the person as physical, intellectual, spiritual, and social. The lived body, in its vulnerabilities and capacities, is a source of human moral wisdom. Although grasped and expressed through the particularities of history and culture and our shared human "nature," our common needs and aspirations indicate boundaries for moral discernment—that is, the forms of interpersonal and social relation, those ideals and practices, that are protective of human flourishing. In a Christian account of embodiment, the human as "spirit in world" is also capable of being revelatory, of expressing the deep mysteries of God's action in human history. Because the human in some sense participates in the divine, biological existence can never be mere "matter" the moral significance of which in any instance is a question of subjective interpretation. At the same time, biological existence has an eternal horizon, which means it is never an absolute value. We will return throughout this study to the question of the "body's wisdom," of what we can hope to know from the enfleshed nature of human reproduction of its social and spiritual significance as well as its malleability, and what we can hope to learn of the contribution as well as the limits of reproductive medicine for the care of the mortal body.

A primary interest in the conditions for human flourishing reflects a second theme or value in the Catholic moral tradition: the embedding of commitments to individual well-being within the *common good*. Concern for the shape and quality of the common life follows from a more fundamental concern for the intrinsic dignity of the human person (as *imago dei*) and the reality of human interdependence in need and potentiality. Because human personhood is assumed to be intrinsically social, human dignity will be expressed, realized, and protected only through membership in various communities. The acknowledgment that individual good requires a rich and protective common life gives rise to both social entitlements and social obligations: all members of a community have a right to a share in the minimum conditions of human well-being and to a basic level of participation;[33] all members have an obligation to contribute to the quality of the common life and to support social, political, and economic institutions that foster "comprehensive human good." The concern for making participation in the life of the community possible for all human beings is also expressed (negatively) in a commitment to address marginalization in various forms (e.g., economic, political, spiritual, physical). So important is the right to participation that a "preferential option for the poor" emerges in Catholic social teaching. A central question for this study is the place of assisted reproduction in a health care system that is oriented toward the common good. In what sense is reproduction a form of social participation? What weight do claims for assistance in reproduction have vis-à-vis other sorts of claims?

Cahill's analysis is useful in showing how we might theologically defend at least some choices to seek assisted reproduction. But there are a number of questions still unanswered. Her careful balancing of the biological and social dimensions of reproduction leaves us with the question of how exactly to honor the importance of embodiment, the physical dimensions of reproductive partnership, without reinforcing the proprietary attitudes toward women and children that have often been associated with an emphasis on genetic parenthood. Cahill rightly avoids the temptation to demonize reproductive technologies. It is not reproductive technology per se we need to resist; indeed, reproductive technologies can be of great benefit to couples who cannot realize a physically generative love without it. But recognizing that should not keep us from questioning those social and cultural forces that compromise our ability to ask the right kind of ethical questions of it. Still, what exactly will it mean to move, as she makes it clear we should, from treating reproduction as purely a matter of individual choice to a matter of the *common* good? How are we to balance an appreciation of the importance of physical and genetic reproduction for individuals and the potential for healing embodied in reproductive technology with attention to its social costs, both economic and cultural?

In what follows, I hope to show not only why these questions are fundamental to our debates over assisted reproduction, but how we might begin to answer them.

NOTES

1 This section draws, in part, on Thomas Shannon, "Assisted Reproduction: An Overview of Technical and Ethical Issues" (paper presented at the International Consultation on New Technologies and Methods of Assisted Reproduction from an Intercultural Perspective, Evangelische Akademie, Loccum, Germany, October 24, 1998).
2 Congregation for the Doctrine of the Faith, "Instruction on Respect for Human Life in its Origin and on the Dignity of Procreation: Replies to Certain Questions of the Day (*Donum Vitae*)," (February 22, 1987) in Edmund D. Pellegrino, John Collins Harvey, and John P. Langan, eds., *Gift of Life: Catholic Scholars Respond to the Vatican Instruction* (Washington, D.C.: Georgetown University Press, 1990), 27.
3 Nicholas Wade, "Embryo Cell Research: A Clash of Values," *The New York Times*, July 2, 1999, A11.
4 Gilbert C. Meilaender, *Body, Soul and Bioethics* (Notre Dame, Ind.: University of Notre Dame Press, 1995), 80.
5 Christine Overall, *Ethics and Human Reproduction: A Feminist Analysis* (Boston: Allen and Unwin, 1987), 9.
6 Margaret A. Farley, "Feminist Theology and Bioethics," in *Women's Consciousness, Women's Conscience: A Reader in Feminist Ethics*, Barbara Hilkert Andolsen, Christine E. Gudorf, and Mary D. Pellauer, eds. (Minneapolis: Winston Press, 1985), 302.
7 Gina Corea, "What the King Cannot See," in *Embryos, Ethics and Women's Rights: Exploring the New Reproductive Technologies*, Elaine Hoffman Baruch, Amadeo F. D'Adamo, Jr., and Joni Seager, eds. (New York: Harrington Park Press, 1988), 90.
8 See, for example, Karl Rahner, "The Problem of Genetic Manipulation," *Theological Investigations*, Vol. 9: Writings of 1965–67. Trans. Graham Harrison (New York: Herder and Herder, 1972), 225–52; Helmut

Thielicke, *The Ethics of Sex.* Trans. John W. Doberstein (New York: Harper and Row, 1964); Paul Ramsey, *Fabricated Man: The Ethics of Genetic Control* (New Haven, Conn.: Yale University Press, 1970), 39; Congregation for the Doctrine of the Faith, "Instruction on Life," 25.

9 Congregation for the Doctrine of the Faith, "Instruction on Life," 25–26.
10 Ibid., 30.
11 Ibid., 27.
12 See Cynthia Cohen, ed., *New Ways of Making Babies: The Case of Egg Donation* (Bloomington: Indiana University Press, 1996).
13 The extent to which commercial relations *actually* enter into assisted reproduction arrangements at this time is in some flux. For example, while a commercial market for human sperm is well established, the trade of human ova or embryos is fairly new. Additionally, the freedom with which persons can accept a fee for acting as a gestational surrogate is a matter of ongoing debate, and regulations vary from state to state. The majority of states have been wary of giving much protection to commercial surrogacy. The moral questions, therefore, arise as much from the potential for commercialization of reproduction through these procedures as from existing practices.
14 Lori Andrews, "Alternative Modes of Reproduction" *Reproductive Laws for the 1990's,* in Sherrill Cohen and Nadine Taub, eds. (Clifton, N.J.: Humana Press, 1989), 361–405; "Feminism Revisited: Fallacies and Policies in the Surrogacy Debate," *Logos* 9 (1988): 81–96. See also, Carmel Shalev, *Birth Power: The Case for Surrogacy* (New Haven, Conn.: Yale University Press, 1989), 146–66.
15 See Lisa Sowle Cahill, *Sex, Gender and Christian Ethics* (Cambridge: Cambridge University Press, 1996); "Women, Marriage, Parenthood: What Are Their 'Natures'?" *Logos* 9 (1988): 11–35; "What Is the 'Nature' of the Unity of Sex, Love and Procreation: A Response to Elio Sgreccia," in Pellegrino, Harvey, and Langan, eds., *Gift of Life,* 137–48.
16 Lisa Sowle Cahill, *Sex, Gender and Christian Ethics* (Cambridge: Cambridge University Press, 1996), 254.
17 Ibid., 252.
18 Cahill, "What is the 'Nature' of the Unity of Sex, Love and Procreation?" 142 (emphasis added).
19 Ibid., 143.
20 Cahill, *Sex, Gender and Christian Ethics,* 246.
21 Paul Lauritzen, *Pursuing Parenthood: Ethical Issues in Assisted Reproduction* (Bloomington: Indiana University Press, 1993): 76–84.
22 Ibid., 83.
23 For an appreciation of this problem, see Cahill's *Family: A Christian Social Perspective* (Minneapolis: Fortress Press, 2000).
24 Lauritzen, *Pursuing Parenthood,* 75.

25 Lauritzen, *Pursuing Parenthood*, 95–97. New techniques for cytoplasm donation would blur the boundaries in a different way. Here, the donor provides cytoplasm, containing mitochondrial DNA, which is injected into the older recipient's egg as a way of "rejuvenating" it. Techniques involving nuclear transfer into an enucleated donor egg would be another case.

26 Thomas H. Murray, *The Worth of a Child* (Berkeley: University of California Press, 1996), 39.

27 Cahill, *Family*, xii.

28 I am grateful to Cristy Traina for encouraging me to develop further the question of adoption.

29 Mary Midgley and Judith Hughes, *Women's Choices: Philosophical Problems Facing Feminism* (London: Weidenfeld and Nicholson), 92.

30 Adoption is often presented as a morally unambiguous solution to infertility, a foil to the morally ambiguous world of assisted reproduction. However, my own experience with the adoption process leaves me unsettled about such comparisons. Like many infertile couples, we explored adoption and, indeed, were in the midst of an adoption preparation class through Catholic Charities when we found out I was pregnant. Although I believe that the decision to adopt can and often does reflect a healthy movement away from the self-concerned obsession with having a child of one's own that underlies choices in assisted reproduction, we should not simply assume that it does, nor should we assume that the adoption process is free of the troubling market values that infect reproductive medicine. There were two moments in the process when I became acutely aware of the irony of holding up adoption as the morally pure alternative to assisted reproduction. The first was when we were given a list of social and physical characteristics of adoptable children and told to indicate those characteristics that would be unacceptable to us. The second was when we were instructed in how to prepare our file to best "sell us" to a prospective birth mother.

31 Germaine Greer, *Sex and Destiny* (New York: Harper and Row, 1984), 481.

32 Again, I am indebted to Cristy Traina for this way of framing the question.

33 National Conference of Catholic Bishops, *Economic Justice for All: Pastoral Letter on Catholic Social Teaching and the U.S. Economy*, #77 (p. 39). The tradition acknowledges that the meaning of "basic level of participation" will vary according to the specific characteristics of the society in which the claim is being made. However, general boundaries are articulated in the form of human rights, the most complete table of which appears in the encyclical *Pacem in Terris*, #11–27 [Pope John XXIII, *Pacem in Terris* April 11, 1963), in *The Gospel of Peace and Justice: Catholic Social Teaching since Pope John,* presented by Joseph Gremillion, (Maryknoll, N.Y.: Orbis Books, 1976), 201–41].

CHAPTER THREE

ASSISTED REPRODUCTION AND THE GOALS OF MEDICINE

"You want to have a baby," he said. "I want us to survive infertility."

—Paulette Bates Alden, *Crossing the Moon: A Journey through Infertility*

During debate on the Unborn Child Protection Bill in the British House of Commons in 1984, one member gave a passionate defense of the aims of assisted reproduction:

> *The object of our interest in medical research into embryology and human fertilisation is to help humanity. It is to help those who are infertile and to help control infertility. . . . The researchers are not monsters, but scientists. They are medical scientists working in response to a great human need. We should be proud of them. The infertile parents who have been helped are grateful to them.[1]*

The extent to which reproductive technologies "help humanity" or "hurt humanity" is, of course, a matter of disagreement. But the speaker hits on a crucial and neuralgic point in the debate over access to treatment for infertility: Involuntary childlessness can be source of considerable human anguish.[2] Treatments that make it possible to conceive and bear children are extremely valuable to those who suffer infertility. But in developing reproductive technologies, in addressing infertility, are we responding to a "great human *need?*"

Efforts to judge the importance of infertility in light of overall medical priorities are often frustrated by the challenge of determining whether an interest in having a child is better characterized as a *want* or a *need*. This distinction can do considerable rhetorical work. Disparities in access to those goods and services human beings *need* are problems of social justice, particu-

66

larly for those who view the world through the lens of Christian ethics. But not every disparity in access to what individuals want or desire is necessarily a problem of justice. Questions of justice or fairness in the distribution of a particular good become more compelling the more important that good is to human survival or well-being.

As we noted earlier, attempts to place reproductive technologies by neatly distinguishing needs from desires are not really very helpful. Our public debates about health care reveal a complex relationship between what we need (individually and collectively) and what we want, between what it takes to sustain our lives and what it takes to satisfy our deepest desires. Except perhaps at the level of the most essential needs, the boundaries between need and want are always defined within a particular cultural and economic context and, as such, are fluid. Moreover, to the extent that reflection about medical funding priorities takes place at all, it is hard to see that it turns primarily on that distinction. To be sure, assumptions about the inherent value of biological life are in the background of our decisions about the importance of life-sustaining treatment. But when we ask if it is wrong to turn away a burn victim in need of emergency treatment or to deny corrective surgery to an infant with cleft palate, it is not first a judgment about whether life is desirable or necessary that motivates the question. Rather, we ask what it means for persons to suffer with this or that condition, what it means to be faced with death or disability, or to have one's life compromised by a certain illness or accident, and what our professional and social obligations are in the face of it.

Nor does it settle all questions simply to decide whether infertility counts as a disease or a disability. "Infertility" as such does not fit the standard definition of "disease." It is not a malady that affects the health status of the infertile person.[3] In fact, as Mary Mahowald points out, "infertility avoids the health risks that pregnancy entails for some women and the discomfort and inconvenience that it entails for virtually all pregnant women."[4]

Yet, as Mahowald acknowledges, and as the courts have at times recognized, many cases of infertility could clearly be called "disability." If by "disability" we mean roughly "a condition that impairs an individual's normal species functioning or usual range of human activity," the inability to conceive a child through sexual intercourse or give birth to a child is a disability in an individual or couple who should ordinarily be able to do so.[5] In what follows, it is this category of infertility I am concerned with—that is, medically diagnosable infertility. But simply classifying infertility as a disability does not get us very far, since it is precisely the question of *what kinds* of disabilities, diseases, impairments, losses, and so on, should fall within the concerns of medicine that presses on us today. We cannot invoke a medical claim for access to assisted reproduction on the basis on "impaired or frustrated opportunities" without having said something about the range of human functions or investments we think it is important or necessary for good medicine or a just society to promote.

A more illuminating way to focus the question of whether medicine should address involuntary childlessness, therefore, is to ask something different: What is the character of the crisis presented by infertility? What should be the goals of medicine today? What is the place of assisted reproductive technologies within those goals? This way of posing the question does not avoid entirely the attempt to discern the difference between "needs" and "wants" or to give some objective value to the experience of childlessness, but it shifts the focus to whether infertility is like or unlike other physical crises where a medical response is assumed to be appropriate. Moreover, it subjects those very assumptions to analysis in light of the debate over systemic priorities now long overdue.

Infertility, Suffering, and the Goals of Medicine

"The warrant for medicine in every culture," argues physician and philosopher Eric Cassell, "is the universal existence of sickness and suffering and the need for relief."[6]

Cassell goes on to make two important observations about suffering and its relevance to the goals of medicine.[7] The first is that suffering is not always a physical state, initiated by physical pain, but can occur in relation to any aspect of a person (the realm of social roles; group identification; relationship with self, body, or family; or one's essential sense of purpose and meaning). Suffering can be described as the "distress brought about by [an] actual or perceived impending threat to the integrity or continued existence of [one's] whole person."[8] Persons suffer "from what they have lost of themselves in relation to the world of objects, events and relationships."[9] Thus, the terminally ill patient suffers as his world disintegrates around him, as he becomes aware that he cannot fulfill the purposes of his life as he has known it. Various losses—the ability to work or to parent, physical attractiveness, sexual potency, physical mobility, freedom to travel—are calculable only in the context of the sufferer's particular life and life goals. Suffering is ameliorated when the threat to self passes or when personal integrity is in some way restored—in some cases by a redefinition of goals.[10]

Cassell's second observation is that, while medicine properly concerns the amelioration of suffering, health care has often caused or deepened the patients' suffering. Care of the body does not always heal the soul, particularly when medical treatment creates or exacerbates personal losses. Moreover, the restoration of wholeness does not necessarily coincide with the cure of illness. Sometimes reintegration occurs only when the patient faces the reality that there is no cure to be had, or when a renegotiation of relationship with the world relieves the anxiety that everything of value is lost or slipping away.

Cassell's reflections on suffering and medicine are important for several reasons. For one thing, he avoids a narrow interpretation of health or illness, in which the terms are only statements regarding a physical condition or the "facts of a body." Rather, in recognizing that suffering occurs in relation to many dimensions of lived experience, Cassell gives social and psychological well-being a central place in any concept of health. He expands our conceptual categories for illness from a physical/organic model to a phenomenological/experiential one, and in doing so, expands the meaning of care. He observes in a later article: "To speak of illness in this manner is to change the habit of mind that sees diseases as natural objects, like oak trees, that are the most important features of the medical landscape, with sick people as the accidental, almost incidental carrier of the disease."[11] When disease is seen as an event affecting *persons* (not simply *bodies*) the challenge of care extends from fixing bodies to recognizing possibilities for maintaining or restoring crucial relationships:

> *The health of the person is a wider goal than the health of the body and reaches into all dimensions of life. The health of the person is the health, not only of the particular individual, but also of the individual as family member, worker, member of the community, political being, and so forth. . . . Success is measured, in this view, not merely by survival or length of life but by function and the fulfillment of personal as well as social roles and goals.*[12]

Were Cassell not so acutely aware of the limits of medicine in restoring health and, indeed, of its capacity to cause suffering in the pursuit of "cure over care," his broad social and relational concept of health would seem antithetical to the goals of systemic reform. But Cassell is not advocating more technology for a wider range of problems—an infinitely expanding sphere of "medical problems." Rather, conceiving health as psychosocial and relational as well as physical is compatible with placing emphasis on prevention of illness. When we view illness as a personal event, we see not only that individuals experience illness relationally but that there are social and relational factors at work in the causation of illness. Helen Rodriquez-Trias captures this insight in speaking of women's health: "Women live in households, communities, and cities and in times, places, and circumstances that spell health or disease, life or death, with greater certainty than does access to health care."[13]

Understanding that people suffer "from what they have lost of themselves in relation to the world of objects, events, and relationships" also enriches the resources we might draw upon for the work of healing. Not only does this account force us to expand the way we think about the problem of suffering in medicine (beyond a physical crisis needing a medical solution) but it encourages therapeutic attention to the possibilities that exist in the family, the community, the health care institution, and the church for accompaniment toward transcendence or reintegration. It also draws critical attention to the social, economic, and cultural forces that impede healing—that is, those material conditions, cultural and religious values, and forms of social imagination of which Cahill spoke, that circumscribe our options for interpreting and resolving problems.

"Suffering" as Cassell understands it does not give us a clear and uncontroversial criterion for deciding medical priorities or for naming entitlements. Not all health-related suffering appears in the form of a crisis; there are those whose experience is not of losing capacities, but of never having had them at all. Moreover, not all losses, obstacles, or threats to self, no matter how much they may evoke suffering, are properly the business of medicine to address. Any conclusions we want to draw about the scope of social and professional duties to alleviate suffering will need to be placed within the larger question of the proper or just aspirations for medicine at this time in history.

Still, in identifying health care priorities, we have to begin somewhere, and it is reasonable to begin with the claim that medicine should have the amelioration of suffering, the protection of well-being and wholeness, as its concern, even though the work remains of discerning where the proper limits of that concern lie. Later we will see interests in human flourishing (as a relational as well as physical value) at the heart of arguments for a fundamental right to health care in the Catholic social tradition. At very least, if we start with an understanding of healing as a restoration not only of bodies or minds but of selves in relation to the "world of objects, events, and relationships," we have an analytically richer starting point for discerning what might properly be asked of a health care system than we will find in analyses that focus on the importance of treating one disease versus another.

How are this account of suffering and the goals of medicine helpful in our reflection on infertility or involuntary childlessness as a health care claim? For those who wish to conceive and bear a child and cannot, infertility is principally a crisis of the self. It is a crisis that can be resolved successfully in medical and nonmedical ways, and one in which medical treatment has often *caused* suffering. It is a crisis that is in many ways mediated by the existence of reproductive technology within a particular cultural context. In infertility, as in illness in general, existing technology defines available options. And it is an experience of suffering that is not easily distinguishable from the experiences of suffering medicine is usually expected to address.

Living with Infertility

Studies of those struggling with infertility reveal some common features of the experience of involuntary childlessness.[14] The realization that one cannot reproduce at will (or perhaps not at all) occasions feelings of grief, loss, and anger; indeed, many infertile patients go through the stages of grieving observed in persons who have received a terminal diagnosis. For those who desire genetic parenting, infertility is an assault on important life plans and widely shared conceptions of the good life. It is an experience of physical powerlessness and loss of control. There are obvious differences between a diagnosis of cancer and a diagnosis of infertility. However, an acknowledgment of infertility confronts patients with the need to redefine personal and relational goals and expectations in a way that shares at least some features of chronic and life-threatening illness. As the normal expectation of growing up, marrying, and raising a family of one's own begins to appear out of reach, so the assumption that the course of one's life is predictable and subject to the powers of reason and will becomes a lie. This aspect of suffering is especially acute for today's "typical" infertility patient: a successful person who has achieved some measure of professional competence, who has carefully executed the various tasks of life, and has now come to the time set aside for reproduction. To be faced with bodies that betray them, or natural forces that refuse to cooperate, is for many individuals an experience of powerlessness for which they have not been prepared.

Because the ability to reproduce is a culturally accepted feature of personal and gender identity, a diagnosis of infertility is often experienced as a statement about far more than the efficiency of an individual's reproductive system. The ability to generate life (or to impregnate) is widely viewed as a flowering of sexual capacity; infertility, therefore, cuts at core assumptions about one's adult sexuality. The feeling that one is a failure, essentially, sexually, and interpersonally, is more acute for women than for men, but it is not unique to women. Many infertile patients describe themselves as feeling "defective," "damaged," or "neutered"; women report feeling "hollow," and "empty," and men express shame at "shooting blanks."[15] They see themselves, not as having imperfect or malfunctioning bodies, but as having spoiled identities. One woman put it this way:

> *I look in the mirror and see a woman who is, in many ways—as a fully freely loving human being—a fraud. I feel profoundly sterile, in ways now that go far beyond the birthing of a child.*[16]

Jan Rehner writes that "when the ability to bear a child is denied a woman, no matter how intelligent, how independent, or how unconventional, she must reexamine what it means to be a woman—not in an impersonal or theoretical way but in terms which strike at the very heart of [her] self-image."[17] My own experience of infertility bears out the truth in Rehner's observation. Having had a professional interest in the ethics of assisted reproduction long before I ever tried to conceive, I was acutely aware of the social construction of infertility, and alert to the trap of mistaking fertility for femininity. But after repeated failures, I came to fear, as many infertile women do, that somehow my body was simply inhospitable to new life. Having always thought of spiritual hospitality as a necessary virtue for the Christian theologian, especially for a feminist theologian, it was extremely difficult, despite all I knew of the "phenomenon," to resist feeling that my infertility revealed not just a disorder in my reproductive system but a defect in the receptivity of my heart. Although the shape of the threat was different, our infertility also forced my husband to confront his understanding of himself as a man.

Studies show that women are more adversely affected by a condition of infertility than are men; women, unlike men, tend to suffer the same emotional reactions to infertility whether there is female factor involved or not; and women are generally the initiators in moving to the next level in infertility treatment.[18] That women experience more stress *during* infertility treatment is understandable, given the fact that the failure of live delivery usually occurs within and through her body no matter what the cause of infertility. Her greater distress is also explained by the reality that examinations and procedures are more likely to be performed on the woman (and are more invasive when they are), and the process of monitoring requires more intense attention to the workings of her system.

But to really understand why women experience deeper loss, pain, and disappointment over involuntary childlessness than men, and why infertility is experienced as a more profound crisis of self for women, we need to appreciate what the infertile woman, "loses of herself in relation to the world of objects, events, and relationships," to borrow Cassell's words. While biological parenthood is a cultural norm for both men and women, the parent role appears to be more central in the transition to adulthood for women than for men. Pregnancy and parenting, as achievements, are still widely perceived to be—and thus are *internalized* as—part of a woman's core identity. The childless woman not only feels judged inferior by the community of adult women but also cut off from participation in that primary community or relegated to a lesser status within it. As Arthur Greil notes, the infertile individual (especially the infertile woman) experiences a stigma "rooted in a powerful sense of failure occasioned by [her] inability to act out a socially approved and personally accepted life script."[19]

Less important for both men and women, but nonetheless significant, is the loss of biological continuity that infertility represents. The human capacity for reproduction serves as both an individual and cultural wall of defense against mortality. For some persons, their inability to reproduce leaves them unable to carry forth a particular family line; for them, to be infertile means to have failed a transgenerational responsibility or trust. One patient described the feeling this way:

> *It was as if a part of me had died, a part of me was never going to be fulfilled. . . . A part of me felt like I was never going to be, a part of me*

*felt like a major disappointment to everybody. I think that was the hard-
est thing. I felt like I had disappointed my husband, I disappointed my
folks, I disappointed his folks, and I disappointed myself.*[20]

For others, the inability to reproduce is symbolic of the inability to do
anything eternal, long-lasting, or transcendent. It represents a loss of the ordinary but profound human power to reach into the next generation. In a social
context where few of our creative contributions will outlast us, where the majority of us will touch the future most enduringly through environmental pol-
lution, the loss of the capacity to contribute through the generation of new life
is especially significant.

As a crisis of the self, experienced within the constellation of interpersonal relationships and values that define a human life, involuntary childlessness often raises fundamental questions of meaning. Just as infertility ushers
in doubt about personal power and agency and the possibility of achieving life
plans, just as it shakes self-esteem and sexuality, so it raises questions about
one's relationship to God and to the deeper energies of life and nature. Infertility renders Sara, the protagonist of Nancy Thayer's *Morning,* invisible: "I
feel as if Fate and God scorn me, disdain me, as if I don't matter to whatever
force it is that brings life into the world."[21]

In some sense the very ordinariness of conception and childbirth is part
of the anguish Sara experiences. All over creation, new life is brought forth
with relative ease and regularity. Not to be able to do such a normal, ordinary
thing, is for many people, a judgment. The force of life finds them unworthy,
or their love as a couple not strong and true enough, or it simply passes them
by as though they did not exist. Whatever the reason, it misses them, it leaves
them empty. The long-standing practice in Judeo-Christian theological and
cultural contexts of speaking of children as blessings, as "gifts from God,"
often intensifies the feelings of having been cursed or punished, especially for
those with deep religious convictions and for those (approximately 10 to15
percent) whose infertility cannot be explained medically.

Many people blame themselves for their inability to conceive. Tending
not to separate a faulty reproductive system from personal failure, they look
to past behavior, previous moral choices, and the often complex reasons they
once gave for wanting or not wanting children in the first place. When was it
that they "tempted fate?" When had it happened that God came to disdain
them? Here, the search for a workable theodicy can interact powerfully with
cultural ideologies and material conditions. Suspecting that the forces of life
have been too harsh or unfair, some pursue the technological solution in order
to defy nature, to make infertility *intentionally* a technical problem. When
natural forces cannot be trusted, it is safer to put faith in science.[22]

The ambiguity of the sexual revolution and its ideal of reproductive control can also play a part in the response of contemporary women to their infertility. When infertility is linked to an untreated sexually transmitted disease,

the effects of an abortion, the long-term use of oral contraceptives, or to a delay in childbearing on personal achievement grounds, the temptation is great to believe that one is merely now "paying the piper," or that God is now exacting penance for earlier sins. Given the connections between sexuality and reproduction, the questions of sin and retribution may be even more acute in this context than in some other types of illness or medical conditions, although they often arise in the experience of illness. Feelings of guilt and self-blame are powerful motivations in the choice to continue with the discomfort and anxiety of infertility treatment despite slim chances of conceiving. The recourse to technology is itself fraught with ambiguity, however, for the woman who believes that "tampering with nature" or the natural order brought upon her a divine judgment in the first place. Does one pay for the past by doing everything humanly possible to conceive? Or is the lesson of the past not to interfere with fate or the forces of life? Reproductive technology is here, as it proves to be in other ways, a mixed-blessing, a means both of gaining peace and intensifying anguish.

What does this phenomenology of infertility tell us? Infertile individuals may not be ill in the usual sense, nor does this condition by itself threaten them with death or physical pain. But we see that the inability to reproduce can be, nonetheless, a source of suffering, an assault touching on all the dimensions of the self that Cassell identified: social roles; group identification; relationship with self, body, or family; life's purposes and meaning. In this sense, infertility represents more than just the privation of the human good of reproduction; it is a failure or impairment of the body that threatens well-being or diminishes the integrity of the whole person. As such, it shares the characteristics of those impairments to health that are arguably the proper concern of medicine.

But we should bear in mind Cassell's second point about medicine as well. It is not only the experience of suffering we need to understand in reflecting on obligations to care, but the interplay of social, cultural, and medical forces that work in defining illness and the possibilities for healing.

Inside/Outside: The Medical Construction of Infertility

Those who want to argue that the infertile are being exploited in assisted reproduction have made much of the "desperation" of the infertile. From all that we have said about the stigma attached to infertility, it is easy to see why the fear of exploitation arises. It would be foolish to deny what is frequently called the "construction of desperation"—that is, the fact that social expectations regarding childbearing work to structure the crisis that is infertility. Yet, there is also a "construction of the infertile patient" (usually woman) that paints infertility as an illness that robs a patient of all capacities for rational or responsible choice. Germaine Greer portrays women who are willing to undergo the rigors of advanced infertility treatment as the "unwitting participants in modern versions of ancient fertility rituals."[23] Renate Klein describes them as so pressured by their husbands and by a pro-natal culture, which stigmatizes them, that they are willing to pay for the privilege of being used as experimental subjects at potential risk to their health.[24]

There is truth in this portrait of "desperation," but it is only a partial picture. Sociological and demographic studies also show infertile patients to be active consumers and strategists, often initially more insistent than their physicians on a need for medical treatment.[25] What is true is that infertile women are usually extremely motivated and many make intentional, self-consciously moral choices, along with their partners, to go to great lengths—sometimes on their own account "irrational" lengths—in the quest for a baby. But the motivations for doing so are only comprehensible at the intersection of desire and possibility, at the point where the deep, perhaps even primordial, impulse toward biological reproduction meets the social, economic, and technological conditions that define how incapacity in the face of it will be lived.

It is a fact of human existence that the appearance of a product structures our perceived need for it. It is not unusual for us to become conscious of the annoyance or discomfort caused by a particular obstacle only when a product is introduced to address it, or to find our tolerance for the discomfort or our willingness to address the obstacle through other means weakened when an attractive solution is now available. It is certainly true that developments in assisted reproductive technology have changed the way infertility is perceived as an obstacle. It would be unfair to argue that interests in biological reproduction are *created* by the development of assisted reproductive technologies, although some have tried to make such an argument. We have already pointed to the deep and complex meanings biological parenthood holds for human beings. Marsh and Ronner's study of infertility in the United States shows a strong and more or less steady investment in infertility treatment, particularly on the part of women, throughout our nation's history.[26] However, it is true that the existence of reproductive technology structures both the definition of the problem of infertility and individuals' perceptions about what would constitute an acceptable resolution of the crisis. It also alters the status of nontechnical or nonmedical solutions.

Medical sociologists point to three interrelated factors influencing the relatively recent growth in the provision and utilization of infertility services. The first is a decreasing availability and attractiveness of nonmedical solutions such as adoption. The second is the rise in infertility among affluent white women, many already seasoned medical consumers. The third is the increased prestige and economic incentives for specialists made possible by modern developments in reproductive endocrinology, microsurgery, and extracorporeal fertilization.[27] It is a good time to be in infertility services because it is a lucrative market where demand for services exceeds supply. Unlike gynecologists of an earlier age, who could offer patients little more than compassion and advice, infertility specialists can now overcome many physical obstacles to pregnancy and, more than ever before, are "miracle workers." Since the accomplishments in reproductive medicine are of high public interest, and the knowledge gained through clinical experimentation extremely valuable beyond its therapeutic applications, a move into infertility medicine can result in a gain in professional status.

The most significant factor in the construction of infertility as illness is the progressive medicalization of infertility. The impetus to find a medical solution for infertility begins, as Marsh and Ronner show, in the late nineteenth century, well before the development of in vitro fertilization.[28] But the introduction of new methods for treating male and female factor infertility has generated a radically new, if not always entirely well-founded, sense of optimism in medicine's ability to overcome infertility, as well as new intensities of interest, not only among medical practitioners, but among patients. Developing abilities to intervene in the reproductive system not only generate new confidence in medicine but deepen the perception of infertility as a technical problem amenable to a technical solution. One consequence is that patients come increasingly to believe that it is possible to effect change through effort. At the same time, patients come increasingly to feel the burden of "not trying hard enough," of not expending enough energy or courage, or of not having had sufficient endurance.

The medicalization of infertility does not appear to be the primary agent in individual decisions to seek medical treatment. At the initial stage, the experiences of role failure seem to exert much more pressure than physician advice or other factors.[29] However, women's experience *within* infertility treatment suggests that once the quest for a baby becomes shaped as a medical problem with a potential medical solution, many patients feel intense pressure to keep going even after their own impulses may have been to quit.

The open-ended character of the infertility crisis accounts in part for the difficulty patients experience in calling an end to the pursuit. Because there is always hope left, at least in principle—there is always another IVF cycle to perform or another insemination to try—it can be quite difficult for persons in long-term infertility treatment to resolve the crisis of involuntary childlessness. Although the course of grieving typically moves, as it does with other crises, from denial to acceptance, in the case of infertility the battle against the condition can be fought over a longer time and broader terrain (the patient is, after all, generally healthy). Therefore, the denial phase is extended. Thus, treatment can make it harder for a person to come to terms with the possibility of never having a biological child or to "face the truth of one's being" that is so central to acceptance. The open-ended quality of infertility treatment also makes it more difficult to redirect energies into other projects or to explore other avenues for resolution.

The significant investments of time and energy involved, coupled with the ideology that effort equals success, can also contribute to the experience of becoming "trapped" in treatment. The "technological imperative" in medicine that others have spoken of creates a continuum of options that seem simply to follow temporally; if one kind of intervention does not work, there is another to which to turn. The longer and more arduous the struggle, the more it can come to seem that only a live birth will vindicate what was endured. Along the way, the physician's interests in a successful outcome can interact with the patient's desire to become pregnant in determining the extent of treatment. Since the course of infertility treatment has no objective failure point, the temptation is great on the part of both patient and specialist to let exhaustion, usually of financial resources, make the call.

To the extent that defining infertility as a medical problem rather than a volitional or psychosomatic problem eases the burden of guilt for persons, it is a positive step. It is also an advance if, by medicalizing infertility, we become more aware of the role of male factors in infertility, and thus move away from the persistent tendency to treat infertility as the woman's "fault." We have earlier seen that it is difficult to separate infertility, as an experience of body-failure with serious psychosocial effects, from other experiences of body-failure that fall within medicine's concerns. We have also acknowledged the practical problems caused by treating assisted reproductive technologies as consumer goods rather than medical goods.

But we can readily see the dangers in the medicalization of infertility. Given a cultural bias toward technological approaches, defining infertility as a medical or technical problem tends to subordinate all other solutions, such as adoption or child-free living, and to circumscribe the dimensions of the problem of infertility. The ethos of technical mastery limits the range of attractive choices, at the same time as it obscures the full nature of the infertility crisis. Thus, while involuntary childlessness is a physical, social, cultural, emotional, interpersonal and spiritual crisis, it quickly becomes just a medical problem, with a resulting emphasis on fixing or bypassing the reproductive system rather than on restoring the self. As we have noted, medicalization is most dangerous when it leads us to mistake the former for the latter. Half of those who seek treatment will have a baby through assisted reproduction and consider their infertility "resolved," but some will successfully resolve the infertility crisis through nontechnical means, some will conceive during treatment but for unknown reasons,[30] and some who conceive and bear a child through artificial reproduction will never resolve the infertility crisis.

The medical treatment of infertility has the problematic effect of participating in the creation and perpetuation of the crisis to which it is offered as a response. Medical attention to infertility interacts with various social forces, in particular with pro-natal ideologies, intensifying not only the alienation of the involuntarily childless but the individual's perception of the condition as an impairment. Procreative therapies are not alone in playing this role, of course. Therapeutic responses to cancer are infused with and driven by cultural beliefs about and fears of death, and the medicalization of cancer can also present obstacles to a successful reintegration of the self. It is hardly just in reproductive medicine that the unexamined drive to cure impoverishes care.

But here Cassell's observations about the importance of acknowledging the limits of medicine in the work of healing are instructive. Medical treatment of the body is an important element in good care, but medicine will not alleviate suffering, and in fact it will be an obstacle to the restoration of the self, if the emotional, spiritual, and social resources for personal transcendence are submerged in the effort to cure or fix the body. Any claims about the importance of assisted reproductive technologies in addressing the suffering that attends infertility, therefore, require honesty about the impact of infertility treatment on the *person* and about the features of reproductive medicine and its social setting that impede the ability of patients to heal, especially where "healing" means accepting limits or exploring alternative options for parenthood. Moreover, any claims about what is important for the care of individuals have to be juxtaposed to the challenge of social transformation—that is, the challenge of transforming the social climate in which impairments or illnesses will be defined, lived, ministered to, and potentially transcended.

Some Preliminary Conclusions

Cassell's rich account of the phenomenon of suffering gives us a useful framework for thinking about why we ought to care for persons under certain circumstances, as well as how we ought to care. Viewed through this lens, it is difficult to distinguish the inability to reproduce from other sources of suffering for which a medical response is assumed to be appropriate. Infertile persons suffer, as do others whose bodies fail them, because of what they have "lost of themselves in relation to the world of objects, events, and relationships." Any description of infertility, that treats it only as a physical impairment will be inadequate. But, so too, will any description of infertility that treats it only as a failure of the social role. The crisis of involuntary childlessness is lived in the space between my inability to realize my purposes or desires through my body and my acceptance of a socially supplied script. It is for this reason that responses to infertility that offer only another way to fulfill the role of parent (such as through adoption) or that focus only on altering the significance of the role (such as by challenging social expectations about women's role in reproduction) are as unsatisfying as those that suppose that reproductive technologies are the simple answer. To care well for persons experiencing involuntary childlessness is to see how physical impairments translate into personal losses, and to ask what among available resources will be valuable in overcoming those losses.

Despite temptations to try, medicine cannot overcome all the limitations of finitude, and good care has often suffered under the illusion that it can. The experience of infertile patients under assisted reproduction supports the observation that more treatment or more aggressive treatment does not necessarily equal better care. If infertility causes anguish because it ushers in feelings of failure and loss of control, modes of treatment that capitalize on those feelings or accentuate them constitute questionable care. Repeated unsuccessful cycles of IVF, for example, which further alienate a woman from her body and plunge her month after month more deeply into the feelings of failure, are not contributing to healing, if what we mean by that is the restoration of the self.

To acknowledge a role for assisted reproductive technologies in ameliorating the suffering associated with infertility does not, therefore, imply endorsement for a battle against infertility at all costs. Good care of those who are suffering involves knowing when aggressive treatment is not called for as well as when it is, and good medicine empowers patients to participate thoughtfully in that judgment. Ultimately, it is the one undergoing treatment who must confront what Jan Rehner called the "fine line between [a] courageous effort to conceive and . . . self-abuse rooted in fear of failure."[31] But the challenge of critical self-awareness is one that has to be brought to reproductive medicine itself, for patients make choices within professional and institutional contexts, where vulnerability and fears of failure intersect with the interests and aims of clinicians and researchers. It is not only the infertile patient's fear of failure that must be scrutinized, but the overall ethos of success in reproductive medicine, not only her potential for crossing the line into a self-abusive obsessive quest for a baby, but the potential of reproductive technology to be tools of abuse.

Reflecting on the nature of suffering is helpful in understanding infertility as a personal crisis and, at least in a preliminary way, in tying infertility to what can be argued to be the warrants for medicine. But arguing that infertility, as a body-failure or impairment, can cause the kind of suffering about which we typically expect medicine to be concerned does not answer the deeper question of the place of assisted reproduction vis-à-vis the aims and purposes of medicine. The problem we face today, at least in developed countries, is having too many human problems for which we call on medicine, too much to offer for too wide a range of complaints, and no consensus of how and where we ought to draw the line. If not every battle ought to be waged, how are we to identify the ones that should? If it is no longer responsible to treat medical care as an individual possession without limits, how are we to think about it as a finite social resource? We cannot be satisfied, therefore, with simply asking what will constitute good care in the case of infertility, as important

as it is to begin there. We need to join that question with an even more fundamental one: What kind of medicine do we and should we want?

Reflecting on the Goals of Medicine

In *The Troubled Dream of Life*, Daniel Callahan asks: "What if the aim of scientific medicine was not an endless struggle against death, with the fight
against disease as the token of that struggle, but helping humans best live a
mortal, not an immortal, life"?[32] Anyone familiar with Callahan's work in
medical ethics knows just how much lies behind the question. For more than
two decades, Callahan has been a trenchant critic of Western medicine's zeal-
ous pursuit of progress, its tendency to take upon itself the problems not just
of disease but of finitude, and to mistake efforts to forestall death with good
care of the dying. More than anyone else, it has been Callahan who has tried
to show that the ethical problems we face today—such as inequalities in access to care, the demand for legalized assisted suicide, and a growing erosion
in trust between patients and health care professionals—stem from a failure to
examine what we ask of medicine and what it really can and ought to do. He
remains in the minority in arguing for age-based rationing of treatment, but
there are many who have come to agree with him that our current problems in
health care require a radical rethinking of the aspirations of medicine—that is,
a "thinking backwards."

The Hastings Center, a bioethics think tank, sponsored a project in the
mid-1990s called "The Goals of Medicine: Setting New Priorities." Spearheaded by Callahan, it brought interdisciplinary teams from fourteen countries, developing as well as developed, together in an international exercise of
backwards thinking.[33] The project report is interesting, both in the level of consensus it reflects with respect to the universal or core values/goals for medicine, and in the obvious difficulties it recognizes in setting health care
priorities, even within any particular society. Its conclusions provide a paradigm of sorts for considering the place of technologies that serve individual
well-being, such as assisted reproduction, in a self-conscious and socially responsible medicine.

Underlying the project are several presuppositions about the current
state of medicine and health care: (1) A failure to set priorities in the development and introduction of new technologies and medical initiatives has re-
sulted in health care systems that are ultimately unsustainable economically
and sustainable in the short term only at an unacceptably high cost in equity
of access. (2) Social investments in health care have not translated into equal
improvements in patient care or population health. (3) Medical and scientific progress has not been guided by a cohesive vision of medicine's contribution to human flourishing as much as by inflated social expectations for

medicine and an ethos of choice. It should be obvious that I am sympathetic with this critique of the status quo. Indeed, it seems that some level of agreement with this general diagnosis would be a precondition to entering into the exercise of articulating and ultimately reconceiving the aims or purposes of medicine.

Any effort to define the universal or core goals of medicine will be fraught with difficulty, of course. Serious disagreements exist, such as between those who argue that medicine has an internal morality, a set of core professional values that transcend its cultural forms, and those who argue that medicine is an evolving, responsive, socially constructed practice without a discernible "essence."[34] There are disagreements as well about exactly how to understand health care as a social resource, whether it is best thought of as a commodity, the value of which is determined by the market, or as an aspect of public service. It should not be surprising, therefore, that we find the strongest consensus at the most general level or that the project's conclusions are often provisional. The report identifies certain core or universal values or ends in medicine: the prevention of disease and injury and the promotion and maintenance of health; the relief of pain and suffering caused by maladies; the care and cure of those with a malady and the care of those who cannot be cured; and the avoidance of premature death and the pursuit of a peaceful death. However, it gives no general formula for prioritizing those ends, either where individual patients are concerned or on the level of health care systems. The prevention of illness and the "care and cure of those with a malady" are given equal status, but no guidance follows for how they might be assigned priority in a competition for resources. Indeed, there is an admirable if ultimately frustrating evenhandedness in treating the various values that are in tension in systemic reform, such as pluralism and universalism, the satisfaction of individual needs and the maintenance of the common good, progress and restraint, equality and liberty. The "middle way" we see is no doubt the price of intercultural dialogue, but it allows for side-stepping precisely at the places where the hard choices would have to made.

The project report is most helpful in suggesting a way of understanding health as a social or relational power in light of which the importance of various social investments in medicine might be weighed. Health is defined here as "the experience of well-being and integrity of mind and body. It is characterized by an acceptable absence of significant malady, and consequently by a person's ability to pursue his or her vital goals and to function in ordinary social and work contexts."[35] As we saw in Cassell, this understanding of health avoids the risk of reducing health merely to a state of physiological functioning and the aim of medicine merely to the continued survival of the body. At the same time, it avoids making health so broad a category that we are no longer sure what would be the particular contribution of medical care to human welfare.

This description of health is not self-interpreting, of course. The report's authors rightly assume that the meaning of "*acceptable* absence of significant malady," "*vital* goals," and "*ordinary* social and work contexts" will be defined locally and dialogically. But we see in it the broad parameters for systemic reform. In general, for example, we could expect a health care system responsive to health as a capacity for acting in the world (not simply as an end in itself) to stress life-enhancing over life-prolonging efforts, to maximize population health over end-stage rescue interventions, and to invest in good public health and access to basic primary and emergency care before making available more expensive care that meets individual curative needs. We could expect as well that concern for the most marginalized members of society would be integral to a system in which health is to be promoted or protected for the sake of pursuing vital human goals or participating in important spheres of human life.

Understanding health as a dimension of the person-in-context is compatible with commitments in feminist ethics to the importance of health care as a means of empowerment. Arguments for including safe contraception and abortion in the definition of "reproductive health" for women, for example, recognize that control of fertility is not only a medical benefit for women and their children, but also an economic, social, and political benefit. The ability to control the circumstances under which one will give birth has implications for women's access to education and employment; by extension, fertility control has implications for women's political and economic standing. "Empowerment" as women's health advocates use it concerns more than just reproductive agency, of course, and not everyone agrees about what is necessary for genuine reproductive agency. The point here is simply that, for feminist ethics, health and well-being have an intrinsically social content and debates over access to health care are part of larger struggles to secure equality of opportunity for women, especially the most marginalized.[36]

An account of the ends of medicine in which success is measured by the ability of persons to pursue important human projects or to fulfill valued social roles is also compatible with the emphasis on the common good that we see in contemporary Catholic social teaching. In the following chapters, I will draw out in more detail the implications of thinking about justice in health care allocation in terms of the common good, and the place of procreative technologies in particular. But it is not hard to see why such a view of health would be attractive for a social ethic in which justice is defined in terms of participation—that is, where individual rights and duties are understood in light of the importance of securing social conditions in which individuals and groups have "ready access to the means of their own fulfillment." The idea that medicine should be concerned, as Callahan puts it, with helping people best live a *mortal* life will also find a sympathetic audience among Christian theologians. Stanley Hauerwas is not alone in arguing that many of our moral debates, such as that over assisted suicide, are rooted in society's denial (and by extension, science and medicine's denial) of what religious traditions understand well: the inevitability of death, the unavoidability of suffering, and the opportunities for grace in both.[37]

Suppose that we accept the thesis that a sustainable and equitable health care system requires that we have realistic expectations of medicine. Suppose, further, that we take the Hastings Center project's definition as a reasonable statement of the core concerns of medicine, that is, the promotion and maintenance of health as "wholeness and basic well-being, the absence of malfunction and . . . the capacity to act in the world." What follows for thinking about the status of reproductive technologies? One broad implication of this view of medicine's goals is a shift in the boundaries of medicine's domain. Priorities that would not be questioned under "cure driven" medicine, such as end-stage rescue therapies for kidney disease, would not be so obvious here, while investments that have been traditionally low priority, such as preventative medicine, would become more important. Moreover, if we understand well-being relationally and see care as a process that allows, when possible, for reintegration of the self, there are obvious limits to scientific medicine's contribution to care and, therefore, opportunities for cooperation between medical and nonmedical parties in the enterprise of care. If this is right, we can begin assessing the place of assisted reproduction by rejecting at least those arguments that presume that reproductive medicine should serve any and every sort of desire for a child or that overcoming infertility requires only medical or technical resources.

This view of the central goals of medicine generates at least a prima facie case for including treatment for infertility in an account of basic care. If what is at stake in social investments in medicine is the ability of a society's members to pursue their vital goals and to function in ordinary social and work contexts, it is difficult to see the basis on which we could categorically exclude infertility, at least if taken, for the moment, on its own merits. It is fair to say that, when it is successful, treatment for infertility restores or compensates for a bodily function or capacity that, while not necessary for daily living, is an important part of normal human potential.[38] When a treatment allows a woman to conceive and give birth to a child, it allows her to pursue an end that is broadly considered a vital goal, a central life achievement. (Something like this was at work in the Clinton plan's inclusion of infertility treatment in its basic benefits package.)

Someone might object that characterizing the ability to conceive and bear a child as a "normal part of human potential" or as a "vital goal" backs into the dangerous connections between maternity and women's "nature" that feminists have rightly criticized. This is an important reservation to raise to the approach I am taking. Given the role of social expectations regarding fertility in creating the stigma under which the infertile suffer, and under which women suffer disproportionately, we would want to be careful indeed of making claims about the importance of conception or childbirth that seem to equate the value of women's lives or the content of human flourishing for women with the ability to bear children.

Yet, acknowledging that having children is widely valued as a feature of a full human life does not commit us to reducing women's social status to childbearer, any more than recognizing that the ability to hold meaningful employment is widely valued as a feature of a full human life, especially for men, commits us to reducing men's status to worker. The danger of playing into social and cultural values that constrain opportunities for resolving losses is real, but the danger of reduction is not unique to women and fertility. Moreover, to disregard the importance of mothering in debates over access to assisted reproduction ignores the value individuals place on the experience of childbearing and childrearing. It is not uncommon to hear both men and women describe their children as the most significant of their achievements. The protagonist of Anna Quindlen's novel, *Black and Blue*, captures this sentiment. Thinking back on her decision to leave an abusive marriage, she reflects:

> *There's not a day when I haven't wondered if I did the right thing then. Leaving Bobby. But, of course, if I hadn't, there would have been no Mike. And therefore, no Grace Ann. Your children make it impossible to regret your past. They're its finest fruits. Sometimes its only ones.*[39]

I do not mean here to romanticize the enterprise of raising children or to suggest that a full human life *requires* having had children of one's own. The point is only that to dismiss the claim that having children is an important feature of how we typically understand a "good mortal life" does not square with the way the experience of parenthood is described in our popular discourse or with the importance, however rhetorical, we place on the social importance of children and the care of children. More important, it does not square with the importance given to mothering in feminist thought. Despite disagreements about the relationship between "care" and "justice" in a feminist ethic, feminists have taken the practices of mothering as morally significant, as paradigmatic of the deep concerns for relationality that mark feminist contributions to ethical and political theory. Indeed, it is not only because of the political significance of reproduction that feminists worry about protecting women's reproductive agency against medical intervention. It is also because of the significance of the event of reproduction in women's lives.[40]

When we recognize health as not merely a state of being or a way of feeling but a capacity for agency, for participation in shared social goods, then the question of allocation in health care is not simply "who is in need?" or "who is suffering?" but "what level of and type of care is needed to enable members of this society to pursue their vital goals and to function in ordinary social and work contexts?" Given both the importance and the ordinariness of reproduction, it seems reasonable to say that treatment for infertility should at least be on the table as decisions about priorities are made. One could argue, of course, that there are other ways to satisfy the desire to participate in the good of parenthood. We can pursue the goal of parenthood, if not through reproduction, through adoption or through extended family relationships. In fact, someone might say, under certain economic, social, and political circumstances, distributive justice might demand pursuing nonmedical rather than medical means of resolving infertility. These are important caveats. In what follows, I explore how we might incorporate the medical and nonmedical in addressing infertility, as well as the intersection of responsibilities and rights in an ethic of the common good. But to grant the possibility of resolving the crisis of infertility through nonmedical means or even the moral obligation to do so under specific circumstances does not vitiate the point I want to make about the standing of infertility in this account of medicine's concerns.

I began this chapter by arguing that the categories of "need" and "want" are not very helpful in trying to talk about the place of infertility treatment in debates over access to health care. Instead, I used the experience of infertility to help us think first about the warrants for medicine and then about the ends medicine ought to serve. Even if medicine's role is only to attend to the frailties of the body that stand in the way of our living a "good, mortal life" we can build a case for including the care of the infertile among its proper ends.

Still, there are several important things missing from our discussion thus far. First, we need some account of human flourishing or human dignity in light of which we can fill out the meaning of a "good, mortal life," and say something about the human significance of reproduction within it. In addition, we need to provide some description of the social conditions for human flourishing so that we have a rational basis for construing the relationship of health care to other social goods and for developing what might be called a "principle of sufficiency," a means for weighing social investments in medicine. Finally, we need principles for defining the scope of legitimate claims against the community and legitimate restrictions on liberty—in other words, for knowing where the limits on reproductive freedom lie or when distributive justice argues against a medical response to infertility.

In the next chapter I take up the question of reproductive liberty. A discussion of the nature of the "right to procreate" does not directly serve the tasks I have just laid out and may seem, therefore, something of a detour at this point. However, the language of rights so permeates our public debates over assisted reproduction that it is difficult to find any treatment of assisted reproduction, positive or negative, that does not turn on a delineation of competing rights. If we are to place our discussion of access to assisted reproduction within the framework of the common good, we will need to get beyond the dominant language of privacy to find a way of talking about reproduction as a social as well as personal event and as a public as well as private trust. We turn now to that challenge.

NOTES

1 Debate on the Unborn Child Protection Bill, House of Commons Debates, 1984–85, 73, column 654; as cited in Naomi Pfeiffer, "Artificial Insemination, in Vitro Fertilization and the Stigma of Infertility," in *Reproductive Technologies*, edited by Michelle Stanworth (Minneapolis: University of Minnesota Press, 1987), 81.

2 "Infertility" and "involuntary childlessness" do not mean the same thing; that is, "infertility" is a condition of the body, which an individual can experience without experiencing involuntary childlessness if children are not desired. I use them interchangeably, however, because I have in mind here principally those individuals who seek treatment for infertility.

3 It is important to note that infertility can be the result of pathological conditions (e.g., endometriosis) that can adversely affect the infertile individual's health status and for which pregnancy could have therapeutic benefit.

4 Mary B. Mahowald, "Ethical Considerations in Infertility," *Infertility: A Comprehensive Text*, edited by Machelle M. Seibel (Stamford, Conn.: Appleton & Lange, 1997), 824.

5 Ibid.

6 Eric J. Cassell, "Recognizing Suffering," *Hastings Center Report* 21, no. 3 (May–June 1991): 24.

7 Eric Cassell, "The Nature of Suffering and the Goals of Medicine," *New England Journal of Medicine* 306, no. 11 (March 18, 1982): 639–45. See also Cassell's *The Nature of Suffering* (New York: Oxford, 1991).

8 Cassell, "Recognizing Suffering," 24.

9 Cassell, "The Nature of Suffering and the Goals of Medicine," 642.

10 The experience of persons diagnosed with the HIV virus who describe finding a new impetus for living (and a new ability to cope) in the decision

to participate in the campaign against the spread of AIDS comes to mind as an example of this sort of redefinition.

11 Eric Cassell, "Pain, Suffering and the Goals of Medicine," in *The Goals of Medicine: The Forgotten Issues in Health Care Reform*, edited by Mark J. Hanson and Daniel Callahan (Washington, D.C.: Georgetown University Press, 1999), 114.

12 Ibid., 115.

13 Helen Rodriguez-Trias, "Women's Health, Women's Lives, Women's Rights," *American Journal of Public Health* 82, no. 5 (1992): 663.

14 See, for example, Antonia Abbey, Frank Andrews, and L. Jill Halman, "Infertility and Subjective Well-Being: The Mediating Roles of Self-Esteem, Internal Control, and Interpersonal Conflict," *Journal of Marriage and the Family* 54, no. 2 (May 1992): 408–18 [a study involving 185 married couples]; Arthur Greil, *Not Yet Pregnant: Infertile Couples in Contemporary America* (New Brunswick, N.J.: Rutgers University Press, 1991) [22 couples]; Aila Collins, Ellen Freeman, Andrea Boxer, and Richard Turek, "Perceptions of Infertility and Treatment Stress in Females as Compared with Males Entering in Vitro Fertilization Treatment," *Fertility and Sterility* 57, no. 2 (February 1992): 350–56 [200 couples]; Miriam Mazor, "Emotional Reactions to Infertility," in *Infertility: Medical, Emotional, and Social Considerations*, edited by Miriam Mazor and Harriet Simons (New York: Human Sciences Press, 1984), 23–35 [100 couples]; Renate Klein, *The Exploitation of a Desire: Women's Experience with IVF, An Exploratory Survey*, unpublished study, Deakin University, Victoria, Australia, 1988 [100 women]. It should be noted that, with the exception of the Klein survey, all the studies noted involved married, middle-class couples, primarily white; samples reflected the demographic profile for infertility services in the United States. There are some variations among study groups with respect to type of treatments sought (e.g., some involved couples undergoing IVF while others excluded those couples), and with respect to whether couples were still in treatment or had dropped out.

15 Abbey, "Infertility and Subjective Well-Being," 409; Greil, *Not Yet Pregnant,* 53; and Mazor, "Emotional Reactions," 27.

16 Jan Rehner, *Infertility: Old Myths: New Meanings* (Toronto: Second Story Press, 1989), 55.

17 Ibid., 53.

18 Robert D. Nachtigall, Gay Becker, and Mark Wozny, "The Effects of Gender-Specific Diagnosis on Men's and Women's Response to Infertility," *Fertility and Sterility* 57, no. 1 (January 1992): 113–20; also Greil, *Not Yet Pregnant,* 51–71.

19 Greil, *Not Yet Pregnant,* 64–66.

20 Ibid., 54.

21 Nancy Thayer, *Morning* (New York: Avon Books, 1987), 164.

22 See Arthur Greil, "Infertility and the Search for Meaning," in *Not Yet Pregnant* (153–73) for an interesting discussion on the subject of theodicy and infertility.

23 Germaine Greer, *The Whole Woman* (New York: Alfred A. Knopf, 1999).

24 Renate Klein, ed., *Infertility: Women Speak Out about Their Experiences of Reproductive Medicine* (London: Pandora Press, 1989), 230.

25 Greil, *Not Yet Pregnant*, 72–104.

26 Margaret Marsh and Wanda Ronner, *The Empty Cradle: Infertility in America from Colonial Times to the Present* (Baltimore: Johns Hopkins University Press, 1996).

27 Greil, *Not Yet Pregnant*, 70; also Rehner, *Infertility*, 75–98.

28 Marsh and Ronner, *The Empty Cradle*, 75–108.

29 Ibid., especially 101–05.

30 One study found that, while 41 percent of couples treated for infertility achieved a successful pregnancy, so did 35 percent of those who had not received treatment (e.g., those on the waiting list). Conception without intervention was, not surprisingly, more common in younger couples. Even within treatment programs, physicians are often at a loss to explain exactly why conception occurred in a certain case. See J. A. Collins, W. Wrixon, L. B. Janes. and E. H. Wilson., "Treatment-Independent Pregnancy among Infertile Couples," *New England Journal of Medicine* (1983) vol. 20, no. 309: 1201–06.

31 Rehner, *Infertility*, 103.

32 Daniel Callahan, *The Troubled Dream of Life: Living with Mortality* (New York: Simon and Schuster, 1993), 189.

33 See "The Goals of Medicine: Setting New Priorities," *Hastings Center Report* 26, no. 6 (November–December 1996), special supplement, S1–27. Also, Mark J. Hanson and Daniel Callahan, eds., *The Goals of Medicine: The Forgotten Issues in Health Care Reform* (Washington, D.C.: Georgetown University Press, 1999).

34 The debates between Edmund Pellegrino and Robert Veatch are a good illustration of this disagreement. See Pellegrino and Thomasma, *The Christian Virtues in Medical Practice* (Washington, D.C.: Georgetown University Press, 1997).

35 "The Goals of Medicine: Setting New Priorities," S9.

36 See Ruth Macklin, "Women's Health: An Ethical Perspective," *Journal of Law, Medicine and Ethics* 21, no. 1 (spring 1993): 23–29.

37 See Gerald P. McKenny, *To Relieve the Human Condition: Bioethics, Technology and the Body* (Albany: State University of New York, 1997) for an excellent treatment of the contribution of religious traditions in this regard.

38 Daniel Callahan, *What Kind of Life? The Limits of Medical Progress* (New York: Simon and Schuster, 1990), 181.

39 Anna Quindlen, *Black and Blue* (New York: Random House, 1998), 369.
40 See Margarete Sandelowski, "Fault Lines: Infertility and Imperiled Sister-hood," *Feminist Studies* 16, no. 1 (spring 1990): 33–51 for an interesting critique of feminist arguments against reproductive technologies.

CHAPTER FOUR

RECONCEIVING PROCREATIVE LIBERTY

It would be funny—if it weren't so painful—how up until about the age of twenty-one the worst mistake a girl like me could make would be to have a baby before she got married, and then almost overnight the worst mistake became to get married and have a baby—both of which I had avoided. I had always been one to want to be in control, never to make a mistake. But now I was beginning to wonder if maybe I wasn't about to make—if I hadn't already—the biggest mistake of all: I was about to miss out on having a child.

—Paulette Bates Alden, *Crossing the Moon: A Journey through Infertility*

Having overheard her mother discussing our infertility problems, my niece—who was about five years old at the time—asked me if I wanted to have a baby. I replied that I wanted very much to have a baby. "Well," she said, "why don't you just get pregnant?"

Yes. Why don't I? Anyone going through infertility treatment learns quickly just how inaccurate it is to call the offspring of assisted reproduction the "children of choice." The phrase, coined by influential legal scholar John Robertson, captures well the popular depiction of "test tube babies" as the "products of will," "made" rather than "begotten," their characteristics carefully selected with nothing left to chance. But for the vast majority of people who need help in initiating or maintaining a pregnancy, the experience of infertility treatment is anything but an experience of having choices and control. If they really could have a "child of choice," most would be grateful just to have a child in the ordinary way. Assisted reproduction is an agonizing waiting game, in which the series of crucial responses—whether or not the ovary responds to medication, the eggs fertilize, and the embryos develop and successfully implant—seem as much a matter of chance as planning.

The rising rate of infertility among older, professional class women is an ironic chapter in the great feminist struggle for women's reproductive liberty. The infertile woman who places herself at the mercy of technology symbolizes at the same time the logical extension of feminist ideals about reproductive agency and their betrayal. For at least some infertile women, their present inability to "have a child at will" is a consequence of their earlier ability to control conception. Fertility once suppressed in the service of freedom, now cannot be recalled. Anita Goldman captures this experience of power slipping into powerlessness:

> *Infertility is the final blow to all those brazen, self-assured, demanding, self-realized, liberated women of her generation. Professing to the world that it is theirs to grasp, to turn, to mould.*
>
> *She took "control" over her body, didn't she, she decided that she should be free to [have sex] without having babies, to sleep with whoever she wanted, without worrying about morals, health, consequences. Then she "determined" she had had enough of that, now she was going to have those babies, now she was ready, mature, self-realized. And then. Bang. Her world shattered. Her decisions meant nothing, her philosophy went on strike, her body rebelled. Against her.*[1]

The ambiguity of reproductive choice is not the only lesson to be learned from our contemporary experience of infertility. The growing number of visits to infertility specialists raises important questions about the long-term safety of available contraceptive methods, the adequacy and availability of preventive gynecological care, and the persistent impact of social structures that force many women to choose between earlier maternity and career advances. But certainly the existential lesson for feminism has been that procreative power, like the force of life itself, is much more elusive than the celebration of control admitted. The alliance between will and body in reproduction is at the same time completely ordinary and remarkably complex.

While "choice" or "control" may not quite describe the experience of assisted reproduction, at least for most people, it is nonetheless true that IVF provides a level of access to the embryo that is not available in "natural" reproduction. By allowing hands-on manipulation of the embryo, assisted reproduction undeniably expands our reproductive options. It is possible to choose whether or not to transfer a particular embryo, or whether to freeze it or destroy it in vitro. It is possible to have one's genetic offspring gestated in another woman's womb. It is possible to select the sex of one's offspring and will soon be possible to safely alter the genetic make-up of an embryo, to increase or decrease the likelihood of an offspring possessing certain traits or characteristics.

It is also true, as Jeremy Rifkin argues, that genetic engineering is a significant "enlargement of human power over life," perhaps "the most advanced form of technics ever conceived."[2] In the service of economic interests of all kinds, genetic and reproductive technologies are powerful extensions of consumer choice. Indeed, the ability to transform oneself or one's offspring genetically makes for the "ultimate consumer playground." Those with resources could always buy a measure of protection from the threat of illness or misfortune. Now those with resources may have the power to alter fate in much more dramatic ways, "recasting [their] own biological endowment and the rest of nature to suit whatever whim might move [them]."[3]

Earlier it was argued that an adequate conception of health must begin with an appreciation of persons as social actors. To be concerned about health is to be concerned not just with the relative state of the body but with the ability of individuals to maintain important social relationships and to pursue valued personal and social goals and projects. From this perspective, the status of assisted reproduction is a question about the nature of genetic parenthood as a personal goal and, in the context of investments in health care, also about its importance as a social project.

The tendency in the United States to treat reproduction as a wholly private matter, to privilege what could be called a liberal rights conception of reproductive autonomy, presents serious obstacles to any attempt to reflect on the social dimensions of assisted reproduction. In an atmosphere where reproductive technologies are often treated simply as extensions of consumer choice, it is difficult to even ask the important questions that accompany arguments for social obligations to address infertility, such as how much and how far? An examination of the influential account of procreative liberty developed by Robertson will prove helpful in showing the limits of the liberal rights paradigm for procreative liberty. More than anyone else, Robertson has shaped the way procreative liberty has been interpreted in debates over the regulation of reproductive technologies and better than any other interpretation, Robertson's account illustrates what is wrong with the liberal conception of reproductive rights. Some readers will see it as obviously deficient on theological grounds. We will see that it is deficient even on its own terms, that it cannot provide the constraints on reproductive decisions its defenders hold to be necessary. Identifying what is wrong with the standard way of thinking about reproductive liberty, we can then begin to reconceive it, to ask how we might understand it as a dimension of well-being within a common good.

John Robertson and the Meaning of Procreative Liberty

Supreme Court Justice William Brennan wrote in *Eisenstadt v. Baird*, that "[i]f the right of privacy means anything, it is the right of the individual, married or single, to be free of unwarranted governmental intrusion into matters so fundamentally affecting a person as the decision whether to bear or beget a child."[4] The presumptive right to freedom from interference in reproduction acknowledges the great importance of reproduction in human life, its centrality to personal identity, meaning, and dignity, as well as the significant burdens of unwanted parenthood. The precise nature and limits of procreative liberty are ill defined, however, and interpretations vary on whether the fundamental right in question is principally a right to bodily integrity, to intimate association, or to conceive an offspring.[5] By expanding reproductive options, noncoital or assisted reproduction further complicates the challenge both of definition and of interpretation.

As a constitutional question, procreative liberty has been affirmed most directly in cases involving the right not to reproduce (e.g., the right to obtain contraceptives or to seek an abortion).[6] The Court has yet to deal explicitly with the right to procreate, in particular with the claims of infertile persons to a right to noninterference in assisted or collaborative reproduction—in other words, reproduction involving contracts with gamete donors or surrogates. Robertson argues that a fundamental right to reproduce through assisted reproduction can be inferred from the Court's protection for privacy in coital reproduction. In the instances where the Court has dealt with the right to reproduce, it has treated marriage and procreation as "among the basic civil rights of man," "essential," "far more precious than property rights."[7] As recently as the 1992 decision in *Casey v. Planned Parenthood,* Justices Kennedy, Souter, and O'Connor observed that "our law affords constitutional protection to personal decisions relating to marriage, procreation, contraception, family relationships, childrearing and education. [These] matters, involving the most intimate and personal choices a person may make in a lifetime, choices central to personal dignity and autonomy, are central to the liberty protected by the Fourteenth Amendment."[8]

Robertson argues that if the Supreme Court can be expected to recognize a married couple's right to procreate coitally, it should recognize a couple's right to procreate noncoitally: "The couple's interest in reproducing is the same, no matter how conception occurs. . . . [T]he values and interests underlying coital reproduction are equally present. Both coital and noncoital conception enable the couple to unite egg and sperm and thus acquire a child of their genes and gestation for rearing."[9] Although he acknowledges the special political problems involved, Robertson argues that protection against interference in reproduction should not be limited to those who are married. Reproductive rights are derived from the central importance of reproduction in an individual's life and require only a capacity to participate meaningfully and an ability to accept or transfer rearing responsibilities. All those who meet the minimum criteria, whether married or not, ought to be free to exercise them.

Because procreative interests are in some instances dependent on the offspring's having certain genetic characteristics, procreative liberty, as Robertson understands it, includes the freedom to enter into collaborative arrangements, to manipulate egg, sperm, or embryo to achieve the desired offspring, and to impede implantation or abort a fetus with undesirable characteristics:

> *People make decisions to reproduce or not because of the package of experiences that they think reproduction or its absence would bring. In many cases, they would not reproduce if it would lead to a packet of experiences X, but they would if it would produce packet Y. Since the makeup of the packet will determine whether or not they reproduce, a right to make reproductive decisions based on that packet should follow. Some right to choose characteristics, either by negative exclusion or positive selection, should follow as well, for the decision to reproduce may often depend upon whether the child will have the characteristics of concern.* [10]

According to this interpretation, a full sense of reproductive autonomy implies the right to control over the circumstances of conception, the conditions of gestation and labor, and the manner of nurture. Therefore, would-be parents (or would-be donors) ought to be free to "separate the genetic, gestational, or social components of reproduction and recombine them in collaboration with others." [11] Founded on an individual's interest in a satisfying procreative experience, the right to reproduce ought to include, in addition to the freedom to alter genetic characteristics, the freedom to choose the sex of the child and to seek the services of another in order to avoid the burdens of gestation and parturition. Procreative rights are not absolute, but "those who would limit procreative choice should have the burden of establishing substantial harm." [12] Claims of harm to society—for example, the concerns about the integrity of connections between sexual intimacy, reproduction, and child-rearing or anxieties about the commodification of reproduction that attend assisted reproduction—are either "too speculative or too moralistic" to justify governmental interference with "quintessentially private choices about family." [13] In the absence of direct, tangible harm to offspring, public policy that interferes with the right to reproduce noncoitally is indefensible.

The right to assisted reproduction remains, in Robertson's analysis, essentially a negative right or a claim to noninterference. While the states can legitimately regulate the circumstances under which persons enter into reproductive contracts (requiring, for example, evidence of sufficient capacity to reproduce, informed consent of all parties, contractual accountability for the welfare of offspring), he argues that they cannot ban or refuse to enforce such transactions altogether without compelling reason. As a negative liberty, however, the right to procreate does not entitle the infertile couple to state-provided services in achieving their interests, on the same grounds that the state has recognized no obligation to provide access to abortion or contraceptives. [14]

RightsTalk and the Critique of Procreative Liberty, American-Style

Robertson captures well why procreative liberty is an important value in the United States. Having and rearing children are experiences of sufficient importance that the conditions under which they occur matter greatly. But Robertson's interpretation of the meaning of procreative liberty in the age of assisted reproduction is deeply unsettling and often criticized. One charge frequently levied at his interpretation is that the language of reproductive "rights" seems inadequate and, in some cases, inappropriate to mediate competing claims and obligations in the context of assisted reproduction. The problem with claims to a right to procreate, as Laura Shanner argues in a 1995 *McGill Law Journal* article, is that they sound too much like claims to objects or material resources.[15] Since what is at stake is not merely the protection of the right to engage in procreative activities, but the freedom to "acquire that sort of child that would make one willing to bring a child into the world in the first place,"[16] it is logical to see the right in question as a right to do whatever is necessary to achieve a certain outcome, in this case, the right to do whatever is necessary to obtain a certain "product." Because reproduction is tied so closely here with one's private conception of a meaningful life, it is not offspring in the abstract that are the object of procreative liberty, but a specific type of offspring—one with those genetic and gender characteristics that will allow it to be incorporated into and contribute to the initiator's overall life project.

At very least, this interpretation of procreative liberty presumes a questionable and arguably impoverished view of reproduction. Parenthood is not so much the undertaking of a project as it is the establishment of a relationship. In reproducing, one does not "acquire a child" but bring into existence a unique and separate individual who, under normal circumstances and through the care and encouragement of the parent(s), will grow into social and moral agency. Focusing on the "unilateral, autonomous rights of the prospective parent," as Shanner points out, "fails to account for the role and status of the child who is produced and who has no say in his or her creation or role in the family."[17] Moreover, children are not like cars or other objects, to be acquired and disposed of according to present tastes, nor are they simply extensions of the self. Rather, while "external to oneself, . . . [the child] is part of an existentially self-defining relationship. . . . Recognition of the child as *an other who defines oneself* captures an [essential] quality of transcendence. . . ." Not entirely one's "issue," still the child reflects oneself, one's past and future; he is potentially autonomous, but only by virtue of relationships of care and nurture.[18]

In this sense, "'having children' is phenomenologically equivalent to 'being a parent,' much as having true friends is experienced as being a friend, or having a lover involves loving. This attitude of transcendental recognition opens up . . . possibilities for interaction, response, appreciation, and understanding of the child as a unique, developing individual."[19] The prevailing paradigm of procreative liberty is deficient from this standpoint in that it encourages an objectifying notion of "acquiring children" over a relational notion of "having children."[20] Indeed, there are some reproductive objectives—such as those requiring the use of genetic screening, selective embryo transfer, abortion or genetic engineering—that can only be accomplished by treating the potential offspring as an object to be created, manipulated, and destroyed according to the terms of the reproductive contract.

A conception of reproductive liberty that privileges the "unilateral, autonomous rights of the prospective parent" has implications not only for how we think about what it is we are doing when we reproduce, but for the treatment and welfare of children in general. Where the interests and desires of would-be parents drive social decisions about reproductive technology, questions about how to pursue the corporate welfare of children—such as what might be required for just reproduction under existing circumstances, whether some arrangements for reproducing are better than others for enhancing the status of children in a particular society, and how investments in potential children relate to social commitments to existing children—have been largely ignored. The National Bioethics Advisory Commission's *Cloning Human Beings* is a case in point. As Daniel Callahan notes, "Nowhere in the report [is there] any reflection on the needs of coming generations of children and how cloning, or biomedical research more broadly, might respond to those needs. There are . . . useful warnings about potential hazards to individual children. . . . There are also plentiful references to reproductive rights, but for the most part it is the welfare and desires of would-be parents, not the needs of children, that are at the core of that notion."[21]

Equally serious is the potential of reproductive rights rhetoric to erode or compromise the primary relationships through which, generally speaking, the welfare of children has been secured. The importance of reproduction to individuals generates the right to manipulate egg, sperm, or embryo to achieve the desired result, to terminate gestation or prevent implantation in the face of undesired results, to enlist the aid of collaborators, and to enter into reproductive contracts for the exchange of gametes or gestational services. What emerges is a view of reproduction in which preconception contracts play the decisive role in defining rearing rights and duties and in determining the meaning of "parent," and in which the only relevant responsibilities are those that are freely chosen. The genetic-gestational-social dimensions of reproduction, it seems, can be severed at will and without cost.

There are good reasons to wonder, however, whether the meanings of reproduction and parenthood or the contours of familial relation are as innocently malleable as all of this assumes. There is no doubt that well-constructed contracts are necessary for clarifying parental rights and duties under assisted reproduction, especially in collaborative or donor-assisted arrangements. It goes without saying that the parties in donor-assisted reproduction need legal protection, although we could hope for much more consideration of the rights of potential offspring than we have seen. However, the underlying presuppositions of "contract parenthood" are unsettling. To begin with, to assume that the preconception contract can be sufficiently clear as to determine parental relationships in advance denies the complexity of reproduction as an affective and social experience as well as a biological one. Our experience with commercial surrogate mothering in the United States suggests that, even if preconception contracts have worked well in the context of artificial insemination, the particular lived experience of pregnancy can complicate the relationship between preconception intentions and post-birth sentiments.

In addition, the nature of what reproductive initiators are contracting about is qualitatively different than the object of ordinary contracts. As a practical matter, it has been difficult to determine the value of specific reproductive contributions and to weigh conflicts between contributors (what is the market value of gestation versus gamete donation?). A contract that may well be sufficient to determine rearing duties and rights with respect to a sperm donor may not address at all the complex physical and affective situation of the surrogate mother or even the ovum donor.

Driven by the professed importance of genetic connection, a contract view of reproductive rights and duties, paradoxically, relativizes genetic or biological connection in the name of reproductive liberty. It is precisely the value of this biological connection, which must remain open for renunciation on the part of the donor or gestator, that justifies the infertile party's right to assistance. Collaborative reproduction may satisfy the needs and interests of the contracting parties, but, as Lisa Sowle Cahill argues, it does so "at the cost of denying the significance of the important dimensions of the relationships they create. While adults may use the arrangement to bring to fruition their own hopes, they create a birth situation in which the child's 'natural' relation of offspring to parent is [a priori and intentionally] impaired."[22]

The intention to assume responsibility for a child ought to be the default condition in any account of "rights" and "entitlements" in reproduction. But the liberal rights conception of procreative liberty has been rightly criticized for going too far in this direction, leaving little or no normative significance to the biological parent-child relationship. At stake is a subtle balance: On the one hand, construing the moral connections between conception, gestation, and rearing in such a way that conception generates an absolute duty to rear ignores what we have learned from the Women's Movement about the importance, both for the welfare of children and the health and safety of women, of honoring a woman's right to decide how and when, if at all, she will give birth. On the other hand, viewing parental obligations and entitlements in isolation from the experiences of conception, pregnancy, and birth treats reproduction as if it can be simply disembodied and as though the conception-gestation-rearing relationship is entirely negotiable. The strong resistance many people feel to commercial surrogacy follows at least in part from an unwillingness to accept the conclusion that a preconception contract negates completely—in either a moral or legal sense—the experiences of having carried and given birth. It is one thing to say that a woman who has conceived, carried, and birthed a child may legitimately choose to transfer rearing obligations to someone else, but quite another to say that this experience of procreation places *no* claim on her as a mother unless she chooses to assume one under the terms of a contract or gives her no special privilege in a conflict over rearing rights and responsibilities.

It may be that our understanding of the experience of procreation can be reinterpreted, as Robertson seems to suggest it can, so that what comes to count as reproduction for one person is the donation of genetic material, for another, the experience of gestation. Imagining a range of possibilities for participating in reproduction could provide a useful corrective to cultural and religious temptations to reduce parenthood simply to genetic connection or to overidentify sexuality with the ability to impregnate or give birth. But, here again, the price of being able to assign various meanings to interchangeable roles is a potential loss of appreciation for the "natural" or intrinsic relation between biological and social parenthood and its setting within the context of spousal love and fidelity. The intense interest of adopted children in finding birth parents or the strong bonds related strangers feel suggests that even if the importance of genetic or familial bonds can be redescribed for the sake of collaborators in assisted reproduction, they may not be so easily redescribed for its offspring.[23]

Just as important, describing or redescribing reproduction primarily in contractual terms, where the meanings of all relationships are open for negotiation, threatens to obscure the element of transcendent commitment that has been an important feature of our understandings of human reproduction, especially in theological interpretations. A central assumption of the liberal model of parental entitlement is that we ought to be free to choose our obligations and to formulate the conditions of our lives to meet our expectations. However, for those faith traditions such as Christianity that value the symbolic or "sacramental" function of the family, family life is privileged in part because it is through familial bonds that we learn to honor indissoluble and predefined obligations as well as the ones we freely incur. The common expression "This child has a face only a mother could love" speaks, of course, to the potential blindness of maternal love, but it also alludes to the "givenness" and duration of parental responsibilities. It captures the ability of a mother's gaze to overlook cultural standards of beauty but also the hope or possibility in parental love of unconditional acceptance and fidelity to children, even to those whose looks or gender or genetic characteristics are not what the parent would have desired or what is prized in a particular society. There is nothing in "contract" reproduction that prevents rearing parents from developing enduring bonds with their children or embracing them in this sort of unconditional love. But neither is there anything in this way of thinking about reproduction that encourages the willingness to enter into reproduction as an "adventure in trust," to accept the undertaking as a relational journey that involves uncertainty, the potential for disappointment, and the necessity of sacrifice. When the presumption that reproductive liberty has its foundation in the individual's interests in a satisfying procreative experience is tied to the capacity and the license to manipulate the elements of reproduction, the enterprise of parenthood takes on a conditionality or tentativeness that cuts against the virtues implicated in a view of parenting as welcoming the other—who is of me but not *mine*—into our midst.

Much of the criticism of Robertson's argument for a broad interpretation of procreative liberty concerns the perceived danger of joining a property model of reproductive rights with expanding technical control over the process of reproduction. Even if not automatically destructive of family relationships or antithetical to the well-being of children, a conception of procreative liberty as the right to "acquire that sort of child that would make one willing to bring a child into the world in the first place" seems to play to the basest temptations of parenthood rather than to its highest ideals. Other criticisms concern its implications for gender equality and its neglect of the ambiguous character of choice in an unjust society. Janet Farrell Smith has argued, for example, that a rights-based or property model of parenting is inherently gender-biased and, therefore, protective of dangerous authority patterns.[24] The concepts of right and entitlement used by Robertson correspond to the values preserved in traditional notions of patriarchal fathering—that is, proprietary control and ownership over wives and children—rather than to those of care and responsibility associated with mothering. To promote a property or "rights centered" model, argues Farrell Smith, whether through vigorous protection of familial autonomy or in the rhetoric of the "right to procreate" debate, is to continue to reinforce an ideal of the family that not only does not encourage more respectful and cooperative parenting styles, but in the past has given permission to the abuse of parental power.

The argument from individual rights in assisted reproduction has also been faulted for tending to trivialize the analysis of means, abstracting the technology both from its social and relational context and its implications. As feminists have been quick to point out, without critical attention to the "who, what, when, where, why, and how," simply providing legal protection for the exercise of choice is illusory and potentially dangerous. Here, as with other arguments for extending negative rights to include women, feminists generally have been suspicious of a defense of personal liberty that papers over inequalities in power or the underlying structural realities of race, class, economics, and politics that will determine how particular technologies will be used, for what, and by whom. As Rosalind Petchesky notes, "the critical issue for feminists is not so much . . . 'the right to choose' as it is the social and material conditions under which choices are made. The 'right to choose' means very little when women are powerless. . . ."[25] If individuals lack the economic means or social leverage to access available technologies on their own behalf, or are subject to various forms of class exploitation as infertility patients or gamete donors, reproductive liberty has not been advanced even if the range of choices one is permitted to make without interference has been expanded. Neither can we say that individuals are "free to choose" when there are no genuinely viable alternatives. If my economic and social resources to raise a handicapped child are small, I am not really able to make a free *choice* about whether or not to continue a pregnancy after prenatal diagnosis reveals a problem. In the same way, insofar as fertility is bound up with self-esteem and social status such that a woman cannot be childless without penalty, a right of noninterference does not guarantee a woman *genuine* freedom to choose or refuse assisted reproduction.

Border Tensions

Whether concerned with the implications of assisted reproduction for the status of women or with the potential impact of assisted reproduction on understandings of marriage, reproduction, and parenthood, the critique of Robertson's interpretation of procreative liberty usually takes, as we have seen, a consequentalist form. Although the case from potential consequences is compelling, it is also possible to show that this interpretation is internally flawed. While defending procreative liberty against virtually all comers, Robertson rejects the frequent charge that he is legitimating an unlimited right to do anything one pleases in the pursuit of a fulfilling reproductive experience. However, it becomes clear when we get to the outer boundaries of procreative liberty—for example, when the rights to clone or to engage in genetic engineering are invoked—that the individual-rights paradigm gives us no coherent internal principle for drawing limits. Having reduced the moral dimensions of procreative choice to individual autonomy and the pursuit of one's reproductive goals, the liberal-rights paradigm cannot provide what the problems of cloning and nontherapeutic genetic engineering call for: an understanding of human reproduction that would tell us why we need not support the right to pursue whatever reproductive goals one happens to have in whatever way one chooses.

As a legal theorist, Robertson is interested in teasing out the logic of constitutional protection for procreative liberty. In suggesting policy directions for regulating reproductive technologies, he reasons casuistically, from reflection on the values at stake in prior defenses of procreative liberty to an interpretation of their salience with regard to a proposed reproductive option. As we move away from sexual reproduction involving a couple's eggs and sperm, the meanings of reproduction, family, parenting, and so on, become blurred. The test of whether a particular reproductive choice or set of choices should be protected is how closely a practice fits with the core "interests, practices, and understandings that make reproduction and having and rearing children a valued activity."[26]

Even for Robertson, some things would-be procreators might want to do seem clearly beyond the limits of procreative liberty. He argues in *Children of Choice,* for example, that creating "replicants" programmed for premature death (as in the 1982 Ridley Scott film *Bladerunner*) or intentionally causing deafness in one's offspring would not qualify as a protected exercise. But on what grounds does Robertson hold that the *Bladerunner* scenario or the interests of a deaf couple in having a deaf child fall outside the protection of procreative liberty? Procreative liberty does not include the right "to create offspring who have fewer capacities than they could otherwise have had," he argues. But why not? If the offspring in question would not otherwise be born at all, and the diminishments are not such that nonexistence would be preferable to existence (as in the case of the intentionally deaf child), what moral objection can be offered to procreation under these circumstances? Robertson's answer is worth quoting at length:

> *Procreative liberty is a protected activity because of the importance of reproduction to personal identity and meaning. When one deliberately tries to have a less than healthy child to serve extraneous goals, the reproductive interests that are ordinarily valued are so diminished that a meaningful conception of the values underlying procreative liberty appear to be absent. Indeed, the* [Bladerunner] *scenario here treats the engineered individual as an object or thing to serve the fabricator's interests, rather than a new person desired in part for his own sake.* Even if no harm accrues to the lesser engineered person (who has no alternative unharmed way to exist) and the fabricator would not otherwise have created a healthier or more whole individual, one can still conclude that the interests and values that underlie respect for procreation do not attach *[here]*.[27]

In the case of the intentionally deaf child, Robertson argues that a couple has no more right to produce a handicapping condition than to deny an existing child necessary treatment for a potentially handicapping condition (that is, to deny the means for future functioning in society). "Unless it can be shown that children born to such parents are in fact better off if they share the parents' disability," stopping parents from "prenatal lessening of offspring abilities" would not "under the view he defends interfere with their procreative liberty."[28] It is the interest in producing "normal healthy children for rearing" (which is not the case with diminishment interventions or cloning) that gives the freedom to reproduce its value.

Prescinding from the question of whether there might be reasons to think that the child of deaf parents might in fact be "better off" sharing his parents' disability, how does Robertson arrive at the conclusion that it is only the interest in producing "normal, healthy children for rearing" that warrants protection? Throughout his reflections on the meaning of procreative liberty, it is the procreators' interests in a meaningful reproductive experience that drives the argument for procreative liberty. Moreover, in several places, he rejects "wrongful life" arguments against protecting the right to bring a child into the world in a diseased, handicapped, or economically impoverished situation. "If offspring are not injured because there is no alternative way for them to be born absent the condition of concern, then reproduction is not irresponsible because of the effect on offspring who are born less whole than is desirable."[29] We might think it morally reprehensible, for example, for a woman to give birth to a child with a withered arm when a brief delay in conception might have avoided it, even if the decision might be defended in terms of the "net benefit" to the child. But if the action is wrong, it is not because she has harmed the child; she has simply "violated a norm against offending persons who are troubled by gratuitous suffering."[30]

Robertson anticipates the question of how he arrives at this seemingly contradictory conclusion: "Of course," he writes in a footnote in *Children of Choice*, "one might ask why only the interest in raising 'normal' children should be protected, if individuals find the same or greater meaning in raising supernormal children [or we might add, 'subnormal children']. At some point a constitutive notion of why reproduction is important has to inform the debate, or else there are no limits to shaping offspring characteristics at all, not even when cloning or intentional diminishment is involved."[31]

But that is precisely what is missing from Robertson's account of procreative liberty: "a constitutive notion of why reproduction is important" capable of generating the conclusion that deliberately trying to have a less than healthy or whole child violates the core values underlying procreative liberty. Having effectively subordinated all other values to the interests of procreators in pursuing a satisfying reproductive experience, he cannot provide a convincing reason, consistent with his position, for why we should object to these uses of reproductive technology any more than to any other. The only notion of why reproduction is important that Robertson provides concerns its importance as "an experience central to individual identity and meaning," and as a means to fulfill important life plans and satisfy desires to transmit genetic heritage.[32] Nowhere do we get an argument for the importance of reproduction to societies (which would tell us why aiming to diminish an offspring's capacities for social participation or other forms of selective breeding might be said to violate core values supporting procreative liberty) or for the importance of reproduction to children (which would tell us why it matters that we desire our children for their own sake).

More important, what is missing here is the recognition of reproduction as establishing what we earlier described as an "existentially self-defining *relationship*" between persons who are distinct however much intertwined. There is nothing in the contract model of reproduction, predicated on the protection of individuals' negative liberties, that explains why it is better to have children (in the relational sense) than to acquire them (as we acquire other goods conducive to the satisfaction of our desires). Moreover, "when liberties, contracts and autonomous agreements are emphasized in pursuing the *objective* of having a baby," as we find in Robertson's defense of procreative liberty, there seems, as Shanner notes, "no reason to prohibit contracts for more specific objectives, such as producing a set of matched offspring [or producing an enhanced offspring]. . . . There is nothing within a contract model . . . to distinguish appropriate from inappropriate activities, nor to promote the objective of forming a healthy family rather than acquiring children as objects."[33] Indeed, preventing this slippery slope in perceptions and behaviors demands what Robertson elsewhere denies but here implicitly admits: that "any contract or agreement be framed in light of values and principles *external* to the autonomous exchange paradigm."

Neither do we have an account of the status of children that would explain why *even if no harm accrues* it would be wrong to bring a human being into the world merely to serve the fabricator's purposes. Only an account of offspring as potentially autonomous beings with a fundamental human dignity would explain why it is morally wrong to treat them as objects or things, or to manipulate genetic characteristics to serve personal reproductive goals. The *Bladerunner* scenario is provocative by virtue of its crassness. But it merely brings into relief a deep social ambivalence concerning the status of children which this defense of procreative liberty leaves unchallenged. Robertson concedes that we are confused about whether offspring are property or persons in the full sense. However, since most reproductive decisions aim at producing a healthy, normal child, conflicts between property or personhood paradigms are usually of little importance, and we should aim to protect reproductive liberty. But the problem of the procreator whose reproductive intentions involve going beyond what is needed for a healthy birth, illustrates why the implicit view of children as property that pervades reproductive rights talk is neither unimportant nor benign. It illustrates as well why an approach to procreative liberty that subordinates all interests to those of the procreator is internally deficient. Here at the boundary, Robertson needs exactly what he has not given us: a way of thinking about reproduction in which the interests of children are integral rather than accidental.

Cloning is a different sort of "boundary problem," but it raises similar problems for Robertson's defense of procreative liberty. Lumping cloning with nontherapeutic genetic engineering, Robertson early on argued that cloning, at least cloning by nuclear transfer, would not fall under procreative liberty. The interests involved "conflict with the values that undergird respect for human reproduction."[34] At points this was simply a formal claim: cloning by somatic cell nuclear transfer may not involve "reproduction" at all if the procreators are not using their DNA or the cells of a previously born offspring.[35] Even when an individual is cloning his or her own DNA, the process may be better described as "duplication" or "replication" than reproduction. We just do not know yet how to place interests in "duplication" or "replication" within the legal and social categories we now employ to talk about reproductive rights.

But in distinguishing cloning from other interventions that aim at creating a healthy, new, biologically related offspring for rearing, Robertson also attempted to mark the boundaries of procreative liberty. Cloning is a problem for procreative liberty, he then argued, not because it necessarily harms offspring, but because it—like intentional diminishment—goes far beyond what is required for a healthy birth. Cloning "breaks the constitutive rules of protected reproduction"; it "deviates too far from prevailing conceptions of what is valuable about reproduction to count as a protected reproductive experience"; it "passes beyond the central experiences of identity and meaning that make reproduction a valued experience."[36]

But, here again, Robertson appeals to something he has not given us: a substantive account of the "constitutive rules of protected reproduction," a sense of what we mean by "central experiences of meaning and identity" in reproduction; a rationale for treating one individual's interest in "self-replication" differently than another's interest in genetic transmission. Indeed, even in suggesting that procreative liberty intends to protect interests in producing a "new, *biologically related* child for rearing," Robertson is forced to qualify his general position. In defending the rights of couples to contract for embryo donation, for example, the desire for a child to rear and the "gestational connection" (which in this case substitutes for "biological relation") had been sufficient to invoke the protection of procreative liberty. Moreover, agnosticism about the meaning of "reproductive interests" gives way to the assumption that procreation entails aiming at a *new, healthy, biologically related* child for rearing. The significance of reproduction is no longer simply whatever the procreator finds meaningful.[37]

Explaining why exerting such a pervasive control over the new individual "violates a basic sense of what makes reproduction valuable," requires mining the very "majoritarian views of right reproduction" Robertson silences in other places as a threat to individual rights. As he cannot in the end help but acknowledge, we recognize an innovation as breaking the rules, exceeding the limits of exception, only by testing it in light of the deeper cultural and religious traditions upon which our understanding of the rules depend. It is hard to see why self-replication should not count as a protected reproductive experience except against the belief that reproduction is at its core a shared enterprise, a partnership involving mutual genetic connection. It is hard to see why the degree of control over the offspring expressed in cloning should be troubling unless we accept and understand something of the warning that children are to be "begotten, not made." It is hard to see why we should count the introduction of asexual reproduction, of the child with a single progenitor, as an unwelcome advance, except against long-held and deeply valued understandings of parenthood as a powerful symbol of sexual intimacy's "two in one flesh" character.

The problem posed by cloning or nontherapeutic genetic manipulation is one of degree, of determining when an intervention deviates so far from "even pluralistic notions of reproductive meaning" so as to undermine the rationale for reproductive liberty. The questions raised are political as well as philosophical, and we cannot hope to do justice to them here, anymore than we can hope to do justice to the complex bioethical questions that attend these practices. But such cases reveal the need for a much thicker conception of reproductive meaning than the simple invocation of individual liberty. It is only by giving voice to the *symbolic*, to particular accounts of the nature of children or the human significance of reproduction capable of calling into question private conceptions of reproductive meaning, that it becomes possible to draw coherent boundaries of the sort Robertson needs to draw. More important, such cases bring home the mistake of supposing that the language of procreative liberty can be detached from the religious and cultural traditions on which our understandings of the core values of reproduction depend and in light of which we know what ought to be protected.

Procreative Liberty and Catholic Social Teaching

If I have described correctly the limits of the liberal-rights paradigm, we are left with the problem of finding a way to talk about reproductive liberty that can take account of the importance of bodily integrity—that is, of not being forced to reproduce against one's will—at the same time as it rejects the assumption that we are entitled to the child we desire. We need to offer a way of thinking about reproduction that protects the ability of parents to raise children according to their religious and cultural values without falsely construing reproduction as an isolated or private matter. The failure of reproductive rights talk to generate a satisfying ethic for assisted reproduction points to the importance of shifting from an individual to a *relational* and *social* understanding of reproduction and shifting from a view of rights as claims against the community to a view of rights as "mutual accountabilities."

The challenge of developing a social conception of rights—a conception in which individual liberty and social welfare are not in necessary or futile opposition—has long been a concern of Roman Catholic social thought. In modern papal and episcopal documents on social questions, we can trace the development of a theory of justice based on a rich and integrated account of human dignity, which presupposes a vision of freedom as intrinsically oriented toward the common good, and which gives rise to a set of limit conditions for liberty in the articulation of a "bias for the poor." As we will see, the failure of the Catholic social tradition to incorporate gender analysis into its reflection on the nature of sexuality, marriage and the family presents certain obstacles to any effort to bring its insights to bear on the problems of reproductive self-determination. However, such obstacles, while serious, are not insurmountable, and enough can be learned from this tradition about the possibilities for moving beyond a liberal-rights conception of procreative liberty toward one capable of taking seriously both the conditions for genuine choice and the effects of choices on the *common good* to make the effort worthwhile.

Dignity, Liberty, and the Common Good

The Second Vatican Council defined the common good as "the sum of those conditions of social life which allow social groups and their members relatively thorough and ready access to their own fulfillment."[38] It is, thus, the "comprehensive human good of all who make up society," encompassing all the spiritual and material aspects that make possible a full and dignified human life. The common good concerns, in the words of Catholic philosopher Jacques Maritain, the "common good of *human persons.*" It is "their communion in good living."[39] It is realized, as David Hollenbach argues, when prevailing social institutions function interdependently for the promotion of, among other things, "strong family life, strong educational institutions, rich cultural and artistic activity," and the "provision of material goods sufficient to meet the needs of all members of society and to allow participation in the civic community."[40]

Based in an account of the human as essentially communal, Catholic social thought advances a conception of justice as *relational* and *mutual.*[41] What is required of individuals, of institutions, or of the social order is specified by the concrete needs of individual persons as they seek to achieve fully human membership in various communities. For this reason, "basic justice demands the establishment of minimum levels of participation in the life of the human community for all persons."[42]

Justice in the social encyclicals focuses on enabling participation for two reasons. First, the Catholic tradition understands the human person as "tending by nature to communion."[43] Our natural desire for relationship or society is a sign of our capacity for self-transcendence, a principle of our perfection:

Persons seek society because as persons they possess an inner urge to the communications of knowledge and love which require relationship with other persons. In its radical generosity, the human person tends to overflow into social communications in response to the law of superabundance inscribed in the depths of being, life, intelligence and love.[44]

Human life is, therefore, "life in community." This is so not only because the full meaning of our humanity is displayed as we achieve union, but because we depend upon the community for the fulfillment of material, intellectual, spiritual, and social needs. We cannot sustain our lives, even in a basic sense, *except* as we are in relation. Concern for enabling participation, therefore, also follows from an interest in what are held to be the necessary social conditions for living a dignified human life. In order for "communion in good living" to occur, responsive social institutions are needed to create or protect the material and nonmaterial conditions under which persons can live together humanly and under which they can develop and exercise common capacities for self-determination, relationship, generativity, intellectual inquiry, faith, and creativity. Over time, understandings have changed concerning the necessary conditions (political, social, institutional, etc.) for a dignified human existence. But it is presupposed throughout the social encyclicals that the mark of a just society is its willingness to guarantee broad access to the "means" of human fulfillment.

The theory of rights that follows from and specifies the meaning and forms of justice in Roman Catholic social teaching could be called "*personalist,* but not individualist."[45] Fundamental rights—to economic initiative, satisfaction of basic human needs, political participation, and religious freedom—are to be protected in the just society not as negative liberties (i.e., rights of noninterference), but as conditions for empowering the individual to contribute to the common life. Since the human person is a "being-in-relation," individual good and collective good are intrinsically intertwined. They are so in such a way, however, that individual freedom, while *oriented* toward the common good, is never simply collapsed into it. The individual and the community can only exist in mutual benefit if individual liberty is respected at the same time as individuals are held accountable to their responsibilities for the maintenance of a good *human* life of the *multitude.*

As opposed to negative liberties, which are self-protective or isolating claims within an existing order, human *rights,* according to this view, are statements about the character of a moral society. As feminist theologian Beverly Harrison argues, in a conception of social justice such as this rooted in a relational-social anthropology, rights designate "the minimal conditions that ought to exist in society to ground personal human well-being."[46] "Rights in a moral sense," therefore, are "shares in the basic conditions of human well-being. [As such,] they are reciprocal accountabilities that are binding for all persons. . . . If I claim a 'right,' I am not only seeking to constrain the other person's action, but I consent to constrain my own in recognition of our common accountabilities."[47] Individual rights, therefore, are relative (modified by commitments to the common life) and reciprocal (they arise in a social field involving correlative duties and counterclaims). Because rights are based on a central principle of respect for human well-being, the freedom of any individual can be legitimately limited or constrained by another's fundamental needs.[48]

Drawing Limits

If "access" and "participation" frame the meaning of the common good, then a fundamental challenge for social ethics is articulating what persons need for participation, or negatively, what conditions are marginalizing. The answers will include more than political liberties, since conditions such as economic hardship, physical suffering, unemployment, and racial and gender discrimination are all factors in marginalization. In addition, there will be ongoing disagreements in any society about what constitutes a minimally acceptable level of participation. This presumes, according to David Hollenbach, an appreciation of the political life as conflictual and pluralistic. But, if the basic conditions for human community can be discerned from a reading of human personality, as argued in the Catholic social tradition, then the "limit condition" for disagreement is drawn by the right of all persons to this "minimally acceptable level of participation."

Where social institutions or policies are failing to guarantee equitable access to the means for a dignified human life, justice will demand preferential treatment for those whose basic needs are not being met. Indeed, for the encyclical tradition, the state of the least well-off stands as a challenge and an indictment to all proposals for social organization. As a principle for directing policy or action, "preferential option for the poor" can be read as having more or less radical implications. In Latin American theologies of liberation, for example, to opt for the poor means to "take up the life and struggle of the poor," to join the poor in claiming what is theirs. For our purposes—that is, for defining the scope of reproductive rights within the common good—it would function primarily as a moral orientation for policy and secondarily as a principle for adjudicating conflicts. As Hollenbach notes, the Catholic social tradition defends an inclusive theory of human rights, both political-legal and sociopolitical. However,

> *defense and support of the full range of rights for every person under*
> *current patterns of economic and political conflict . . . [call] for a*
> *choice. This choice is one that will orient policy toward preferential con-*
> *cern for the rights of those who have neither bread nor freedom. It*
> *means that rights of the oppressed, those denied both political and*

> *economic power, should take priority in policy over privileged forms of influence and wealth.*[49]

Opting for the poor, therefore, entails the responsibility to evaluate social policy from the perspective of those who are variously marginalized within the present order as well as a commitment to unseating unjust patterns of privilege within it, even at some cost to the liberty of the now privileged.[50]

We have said that the Catholic social tradition yields an analytical framework where self-determination and the common good are not in necessary or futile opposition. But it is obvious when we take up the question of the poor that that does not mean that these values are never in conflict. Indeed, the problems of distributive justice in health care with which we are dealing here involve just such conflicts and on several different levels. It does mean that the tensions between respecting self-determination and promoting social accountability cannot be resolved in a simple choice of one *over* the other. The challenge of addressing dehumanizing living conditions or gross disparities in economic power or political voice is not simply a matter of "changing who is on top."[51] It involves examining social, economic, political, and cultural institutions and practices in light of the general requirements of human flourishing, chief among which is the capacity for moral agency. At stake in "opting for the poor" is the inclusion of those who have been marginalized in an order oriented toward human development in common, not the substitution of a different kind of marginalization for what now exists. At the same time, to seek the *common* good means that no individual or group can argue for the protection of rights or liberties which can only be maintained by denying the fundamental rights of others.

Situating Procreative Liberty

In chapter 5, we will take up directly the questions of distributive justice that arise in the context of assisted reproduction. There we will ask how we ought to judge the importance of guaranteeing access to infertility treatment in light of commitments to protecting a "decent and equitable level of access" to the goods needed to meet basic human needs. But I have argued that the Catholic social tradition gives us a way of thinking about rights that makes the relationship between freedom and accountability intrinsic, a way that allows us to imagine claims against the community that are not simply individualistic. What, then, can be learned from thinking about reproductive rights in this way, as, in Harrison's words, "shares in the minimum conditions of human well-being"?

Procreative rights are a good illustration both of the interrelation between rights and duties in the Catholic tradition and the interplay of social, economic, and political rights. Procreation is a natural right, preceding the state, but entailing duties that can be satisfied only in a protective and empowering social environment.[52] The right to procreate follows from the nature of the person, in the principle of generativity that is part of the tradition's description of the human *telos*. For this reason, procreative liberty must be acknowledged by the state, but cannot be granted by it. However, the right to procreate presupposes the obligation to assume responsibility for the care and education of offspring. Because carrying out those duties requires specific kinds of social support, the state has an obligation to protect the conditions under which the freedom to choose a state in life and to bear and rear children can be exercised with dignity. In a sense, therefore, the right to procreate has both negative and positive dimensions in Catholic social thought. It is a right of noninterference insofar as the meaning of respect for bodily integrity includes not being prevented from realizing procreation and parenthood as a basic element of physical flourishing. But choice here is not, as Martha Nussbaum put it, "pure spontaneity, flourishing independently of material and social conditions."[53] Genuine procreative liberty depends upon a guarantee of the "conditions of possibility" for its responsible exercise. Thus the right to procreate intersects with other economic and social rights that are claims to certain minimum conditions for exercising the rights and fulfilling the duties that are attached—for example, the right to a living wage and the broader right to economic development.

For the Catholic social tradition, procreative liberty is more than a grant of permission. It is the existence of social, economic, and interpersonal conditions that make reproduction possible as a fitting human act. In principle, therefore, procreative liberty so understood contains its own constraints. For example, since human dignity is the foundation for obligations to the common good, duties to respect the fundamental dignity of offspring (as potentially autonomous, and possessing certain physical, intellectual, and spiritual capacities) count against any individual's right, to paraphrase Robertson, to acquire a child that meets his or her reproductive specifications. Reproduction is inherently relational, "other-regarding," not just in a physical sense but a moral sense. To reproduce is to welcome a new being with equal rights, qua human being, to the basic means for human development.[54] To reproduce is to incur obligations to act so as to protect the conditions for human flourishing on behalf of the one who has come into your care. Reproductive liberty, therefore, presupposes both the willingness and the ability to provide for the physical, social, and spiritual needs of offspring. It also presupposes obligations to respect the equal rights of the offspring, such as the right to respect for his or her fundamental human uniqueness. Some sense of this is behind arguments against a parental license on genetic engineering. The right to an "open future," as it is often called is the right to respect for one's given and particular genetic destiny.

Because consistency and intimacy in nurture contribute to the development of intellectual and emotional capacities in children, there are good reasons to question reproductive practices that detach interests in creating offspring from commitments to care for them or social policies that undermine the ability of those adults most closely concerned to act on a child's behalf. Respect for human dignity takes concrete shape in concern for equitable access to the means for social participation. Therefore, reproductive responsibility includes questioning reproductive practices that reinforce social patterns of discrimination, such as sex preselection and certain forms of reproductive eugenics. In addition, placing reproductive liberty in the context of the common good entails examining the impact of reproductive behaviors on the social "conditions of possibility" for humane reproduction. It is not only possible but it is necessary to ask how recourse to assisted reproductive technologies promises to enhance or diminish the potential for experiencing reproduction as a fitting human act and how reproductive choice relates to other elements of reproductive self-determination, such as the availability of attractive alternatives to maternity or the provision of basic health care.

The promise of such an account of procreative liberty for drawing potential limits for reproductive choice, however, is not fully realized in the Catholic social tradition. The population question provides the best illustration. We saw that the individual and common good are said to exist in a relationship of mutual implication. Social conditions should facilitate individual flourishing, and the common good is achieved when the dignity of individuals as "agents of their own lives" is guaranteed. For this reason population control programs that systematically take reproductive choice away from individuals or that render them objects rather than subjects of policy have been vigorously opposed. Although the Church has acknowleged that global population pressures exist, it has consistently argued that demographic problems are problems of power, control, and greed which require political and economic restructuring.[55] A just society has an obligation to make possible the means—a decent wage, health, shelter, environmental security—necessary for carrying out the responsibilities of parenthood. Couples have an obligation to take familial, social, and economic factors into consideration in making choices concerning reproduction. However, the obligations of responsible reproduction do not run all the way in the other direction. Social or relational conditions can never impose an obligation on the couple to *avoid* procreation.[56]

There are at least two reasons why social accountability takes the form of a permission to limit reproduction and never an obligation. First, moral limits on the scope of reproductive choice follow from what is held to be the objective structure of the conjugal act. Procreation is not only a basic human good, but a duty that follows from the nature of the marriage relationship. The right to procreate is not a right, once again, that can be granted by the state (or, therefore, rescinded) nor one that resides in individuals. It is a natural right one has *through* one's spouse.[57] Decisions to exercise control over fertility must be made in such a way as to respect the natural *telos* of the sexual act, its proper setting in marriage, and its intrinsic reproductive finality. No one can be morally required to act in violation of the ends either of sexual intercourse or of marriage.

A further reason why reproductive accountability does not have the same force as reproductive autonomy is the Catholic social tradition's tendency to privatize the family or relegate it to the "natural" realm. While, for example, contemporary papal documents uphold what they interpret as the essential equality of men and women, they also presuppose a divinely ordained gendered differentiation and complementarity of roles. Despite a gradual recognition by the popes of situations of social inequality between men and women, and a commitment in more recent papal documents to encouraging greater participation by women in the public sphere, the language about women's service to the community has consistently presupposed an essentially "private," domestic, even reproductive vocation.[58] John Paul II, while arguing that "the equal dignity and responsibility of men and women fully justifies women's access to public functions," nonetheless reminded his readers that "the true advancement of women requires that clear recognition be given to the value of their maternal and family role, by comparison with all other public roles and all other professions."[59] One consequence of translating equality into complementarity is that the commitments of the Catholic tradition regarding equality, self-determination, access, and justice in society, etc., are not visible in its assessment of the family.[60] A further consequence is that the tradition fails to recognize genuine conflicts between the goods of reproduction and access (especially for women) to the means for full human flourishing.

Many Catholic theologians have argued for a richer, more integrated theology of human sexuality.[61] Without denying the symbolic significance of sexual reproduction, they call into question the assumption that the entire moral content of sexual intercourse is contained in its objective structure. Rather, they have argued that sexual expression is a complex language, the moral evaluation of which depends upon various features of the encounter, such as the uses of power involved, the level of responsibility for consequences accepted by the parties, the presumption of mutuality and consent, and the degree of authenticity of desire. To separate sexual expression and reproduction does not violate the moral meaning of sexuality. Indeed, the ability to do so is in some sense a precondition for responsibility in sexual expression.

Many people share the Vatican's opposition to forced choices concerning reproduction. A growing international consensus has identified the education of women (and, by extension, improvements in the status of women) as the primary factor in reducing dangerous population trends, far more important than access to contraceptives. At the same time, the means to determine the circumstances under which one will reproduce have a direct relationship to the ability to pursue intellectual and personal growth and civic involvement, and therefore, a relationship to overall gains in women's status. It has become increasingly clear that the ability to have genuine control over reproduction is a critical component in women's development and opportunity for social participation. Especially in areas where a woman's social status is determined by her fertility, the creation of conditions where she can responsibly decide *not* to procreate (that is, where women have economic security, adequate health care, sexual education, etc.) is as important to procreative liberty as a dimension of human flourishing as the creation of conditions for permitting responsible reproduction.

But moral considerations go even further. However, to realize the full implications of placing reproductive liberty within a concern for the common good, we need to consider the possibility of moral obligations to avoid procreation. If it makes sense to think of rights as "mutual accountabilities," and to argue that we have no claim to forms of liberty that can only be maintained at the price of others' basic or survival needs, we can imagine a moral constraint on individual choices to reproduce under conditions, for example, where population pressures undermine social, economic, and ecological stability or where reproduction for some can only be accomplished by denying others access to some basic human good, such as health care. To recognize an obligation under some circumstances to refrain from reproduction does not require us to accept birth quotas or other government-imposed birth regulation policies. There are ample ethical and practical reasons for thinking that top-down approaches are not the best way to address questions of social accountability in reproduction. The point is simply that if we are to bring the Catholic social tradition's reflection on the demands of justice to bear on the family and its relationship to the common good, there is no special amnesty for choices about reproduction. Just as a concern for the common good places what John Paul II called a "social mortgage" on choices concerning private property, so should that concern place expectations of accountability on reproductive decisions. When and how moral pressure might be brought to bear with regard to reproductive choice is a complex question which can only be answered locally, in the context of specific social, economic, and political realities. When and how moral pressure ought to be brought to bear on choices within assisted reproduction is an even more complex questions that we will make some attempt to answer in the next chapter. But it seems clear that to fully bring a social and relational concept of rights to bear on reproductive choice we need to be willing to acknowledge not only *internal* limits, in the form of respect for the dignity of the potential offspring, but *external* limits, in the form of obligations to assess the impact on reproductive decisions on the social fabric and to refrain under some circumstances.

Conclusion

In this chapter, we have offered a way to think about procreative liberty that takes us beyond the liberal-rights paradigm that governs debate over reproductive rights today. By understanding rights as shares in the minimum conditions of human well-being, it is possible to incorporate an appreciation of the importance of the capacity to reproduce as a dimension of human flourishing without ignoring the social effects of reproductive choices. In principle, efforts to find adequate and compassionate responses to infertility, whether through technology or some other means, need not be opposed to but can be part of the goal of creating social conditions for responsible human reproduction. Since the common good pertains to the good of human persons, the social and interpersonal conditions that permit meaningful participation will serve basic physical, emotional, spiritual, and intellectual well-being.

Social justice, for a Catholic social ethic, acknowledges that "persons have an obligation to be active and productive participants in the life of society and that society has a duty to enable them to participate in this way."[62] Previously I have argued for an account of the goals of medicine that links access to health care with social agency. I have also tried to isolate the features of infertility that place it within medicine's concerns for the physical and relational aspects of human flourishing. But the question remains of how exactly to assess the importance of access to treatment for infertility in light of social obligations to secure what could be called a "floor of well-being" or to satisfy basic human needs. How are we to judge the importance of assisted reproduction for the infertile against other kinds of medical and nonmedical goods when claims compete? Given constraints in health care spending and serious problems of access, where should the limits to technological assistance in the pursuit of parenthood be drawn? Given concerns for human dignity that underlie a commitment to the common good, are there some forms of assisted reproduction that fail to meet the tests of justice, even if they can be provided fairly? Questions of just allocation in health care well may be, in the end, irresolvable, as Paul Ramsey long ago observed. But even if we will not solve them to everyone's satisfaction, they are the point to which we have naturally come, and to them we now turn.

NOTES

1 Anita Goldman, "The Production of Eggs and the Will of God," in Renate Klein, ed., *Infertility: Women Speak Out about Their Experiences of Reproductive Medicine* (London: Pandora Press, 1989), 73.

2 Jeremy Rifken, *The Biotech Century* (New York: Tarcher-Putnam, 1998), 226.

3 Ibid.

4 405 U.S. 438, 453 (1972). *Eisenstadt v. Baird* held that the privacy right to contraception extends to unmarried individuals.

5 This is because privacy rights are invoked to protect the liberty to enter into a marriage, to bear and rear offspring, to purchase and use contraception, to refuse enforced sterilization, and to terminate a pregnancy under certain conditions. These involve, obviously, different senses of "privacy."

6 See *Griswold v. Connecticut,* 381 U.S. 479 (1965); *Eisenstadt v. Baird,* 405 U.S. 438 (1972); *Roe v. Wade,* 410 U.S. 113 (1973).

7 *Stanley v. Illinois,* 405 U.S. 645, 651 (1972); also, *Skinner v. Oklahoma,* 316 U.S. 535, 541 (1942); *Meyer v. Nebraska,* 262 U.S. 390, 393 (1923); *Cleveland Board of Education v. LaFleur,* 414 U.S. 632, 639–40 (1973). Also, John Robertson, "Procreative Liberty and the Control of Conception, Pregnancy, and Childbirth, *Virginia Law Review* 69 (1983): 405.

8 *Casey v. Planned Parenthood,* 112 S. Ct. 2791 (1992) as quoted in John Robertson, *Children of Choice: Freedom and the New Reproductive Technologies* (Princeton, N.J.: Princeton University Press, 1994), 37.

9 John Robertson, "Embryos, Families, and Procreative Liberty: The Legal Structure of the New Reproduction" *Southern California Law Review* 59 (1986): 939, 961.

10 John Robertson, "Liberty, Identity, and Human Cloning," *Texas Law Review* 76 (1998): 1371, 1390–91.

116

11 Robertson, "Procreative Liberty," 410; and "Embryos, Families, and Procreative Liberty," 961–62.

12 Robertson, *Children of Choice,* 40–41.

13 Robertson, "Liberty, Identity, and Human Cloning," 1371.

14 Robertson argues that while religious or cultural concerns about sexuality, reproduction, female roles, etc., are not unimportant in decisions regarding the use of procreative technologies, they do not justify public restrictions on access. He writes, "There is no way to understand cases such as *Roe v. Wade, Eisenstadt v. Baird, Griswold v. Connecticut,* and a host of others other than as standing for the proposition that symbolic or moral evaluation of protected conduct without more does not justify state interference with the conduct. The community's power to enforce or impose morality stops at the threshold of another person's fundamental rights." Moral or symbolic concerns may, however, justify the state's refusal to fund certain reproductive activities, as in the case of abortion (John Robertson, "Embryos, Families, and Procreative Liberty," 966, fn. 82).

15 Laura Shanner, "The Right to Procreate: When Rights Claims Have Gone Wrong," *McGill Law Journal* 40 (1995): 823–874, 859.

16 Robertson, "Procreative Liberty," 69, 405, 432.

17 Shanner, *The Right to Procreate,* 858.

18 Ibid., 859.

19 Ibid.

20 A similar argument is made by Oliver O'Donovan and Gilbert Meilaender on theological grounds. The religious language of "begetting" captures this sense of an otherness and distinctive nature of the child, who is received in trust but never possessed. As Meilaender writes: "Our children begin with a kind of genetic independence of us, their parents. They replicate neither their father nor their mother. That is a reminder of the independence that we must eventually grant to them and for which it is our duty to prepare them" (in "Begetting and Cloning" *First Things* [June–July 1997]: 41, 42).

21 Daniel Callahan, "Cloning: The Work Not Done," *Hastings Center Report* 27, no. 5 (1997): 19.

22 Lisa Sowle Cahill, "Moral Traditions, Ethical Languages," *Journal of Medicine and Philosophy* 14, no. 5 (1990): 519.

23 There is not as yet a consensus on the long-range psychological effects of donor-assisted reproduction on offspring. Studies of donor-assisted artificial insemination have demonstrated negative effects from the practice of secrecy, and some surveys of adults who identify themselves as having been conceived through donor-assisted insemination show them to be highly interested in meeting their anonymous donor. But it is not clear yet to what degree the psychological features of donor-egg and surrogacy will be like or unlike the psychological features of adoption, or what practices

(e.g., of disclosure) will be important in minimizing negative consequences of such methods.

24 Janet Farrell Smith, "Parenting and Property," in *Mothering: Essays in Feminist Theory*, Joyce Treblicott, ed. (Totowa, N.J.: Rowman and Allan-held, 1983), 199–210.

25 Rosalind P. Petchesky, "Reproductive Freedom: Beyond 'A Woman's Right to Choose,'" *Journal of Women in Culture and Society* 5 (1979): 674.

26 Robertson, "Liberty, Identity, and Human Cloning," 1392.

27 Robertson, *Children of Choice*, 171 (emphasis in Roman type added).

28 Ibid., 171. See also 169. Emphasis added.

29 Ibid., 76.

30 Ibid. The case to which he is referring is drawn from Derek Parfit, "On Doing the Best for Our Children," in *Ethics and Population*, edited by M. D. Bayles (Cambridge: Schenkman, 1976).

31 Ibid., 263, fn. 40.

32 Ibid., 24.

33 Shanner, "The Right to Procreate," 862, fn. 19.

34 Robertson, *Children of Choice,* 172. In subsequent writings, Robertson in-cludes cloning by nuclear transfer under the umbrella of procreative lib-erty. See "Liberty, Identity, and Human Cloning." But, as many have pointed out, the rationale for his shift is not clear.

35 Elsewhere, he treats cloning by blastomere separation as simply an exten-sion of procreative liberty. See "The Question of Human Cloning," *Hastings Center Report* 24, no. 2 (March–April, 1994): 6.

36 Robertson, *Children of Choice*, 169.

37 Ibid., 32.

38 Pope Paul VI, *Gaudium et Spes* (1965), #26, as cited in National Confer-ence of Catholic Bishops, *Economic Justice for All: Pastoral Letter on Catholic Social Teaching and the U.S. Economy* (Washington, D.C.: Na-tional Conference of Catholic Bishops/United States Catholic Conference, 1986), #79.

39 Jacques Maritain, *The Person and the Common Good* (Notre Dame, Ind.: Notre Dame University Press), 50 (originally published in 1946).

40 David Hollenbach, "Liberalism, Communitarianism, and the Bishops' Pastoral Letter on the Economy," *Annual of the Society of Christian Ethics* (1987): 27.

41 I am indebted here to Hollenbach's interpretation of justice in Roman Catholic social thought. See David Hollenbach, *Justice, Peace, and Human Rights* (New York: Crossroad, 1988), 16–33; "The Common Good Revis-ited," *Theological Studies* 50, no. 1 (1989): 83–84; and "Liberalism, Com-munitarianism, and the Bishops' Pastoral Letter on the Economy," *Annual of the Society of Christian Ethics* (1987): 19–53. For further commentary on the role of a relational anthropology in Roman Catholic social thought,

see Jean-Yves Calvez, S.J., and Jacques Perrin, S.J., *The Church and Social Justice: The Social Teaching of the Popes from Leo XIII to Pius XII (1878–1958),* (Chicago: Henry Regnery Co., 1961), 101–33; Daniel A. O'Connor, C.S.V., *Catholic Social Doctrine* (Westminster, England: The Newman Press, 1956), 149–59; Ernie Cortes, "Reflections on the Catholic Tradition of Family Rights," and Charles E. Curran, "Catholic Social Teaching and Human Morality," in *One Hundred Years of Catholic Social Thought,* edited by John A. Coleman, S.J. (Maryknoll, N.Y.: Orbis Books, 1991), 160–62; 74–80; Michael J. Schuck, *That They Be One: The Social Teaching of the Papal Encyclicals, 1740–1989* (Washington, D.C.: Georgetown University Press, 1991), 173–90.

42 National Conference of Catholic Bishops, *Economic Justice for All,* 39–40.

43 Maritain, *The Person and the Common Good,* 47. Maritain is not only a helpful interpreter of the theological and philosophical roots of Roman Catholic social thought but an influential figure in its development.

44 Ibid., 47–48.

45 David Hollenbach, *Claims in Conflict: Retrieving and Renewing the Catholic Human Rights Tradition* (New York: Paulist Press, 1979), 97 (emphasis added).

46 Beverly Wildung Harrison, *Our Right to Choose: Toward a New Ethic of Abortion* (Boston: Beacon Press, 1983), 197 (emphasis added).

47 Ibid.

48 See Beverly Wildung Harrison,"Theological Reflection in the Struggle for Liberation," in *Making the Connections,* Carol S. Robb, ed. (Boston: Beacon Press, 1985), 225.

49 Hollenbach, *Justice, Peace and Human Rights,* 99.

50 There are various interpretations of "option for" or "bias for" the poor within the tradition, some of which would support a stronger statement than others of the limits that might be placed on the liberty of the well-off for the sake of the poor. In *Centesimus Annus,* John Paul seems to back off the more radical interpretations of "bias," arguing that option for the poor is never "exclusive or discriminatory toward other groups," [John Paul II, *Centesimus Annus* (May 1, 1991), #57, reprinted in *National Catholic Reporter,* May 24, 1991, p. 29)]. See also Pope John Paul II, *Sollicitudo Rei Socialis,* #39 (December 30, 1987) in *Origins* 17, no. 38 (March 3, 1988), 654. But his qualification here is not always consistent with other arguments in his social encyclicals concerning the "social mortgage" on rights such as private property.

51 Some have argued that violent revolution in the Christian tradition is justified as vindication for the rights of the poor. However, I think it can be shown that any resolution to the great gaps between rich and poor that simply overturns the present order for a different sort of oppressive order

misses the spirit of the Catholic social tradition. See Donal Dorr, *Option for the Poor: A Hundred Years of Vatican Social Teaching* (Maryknoll, N.Y.: Orbis Books, 1983) for a historical study of the development of the doctrine of preferential option.

52 Pope John XXIII, *Pacem in Terris,* April 11, 1963, #15, in *The Gospel of Peace and Justice: Catholic Social Teaching since Pope John,* presented by Joseph Gremillion (Maryknoll, N.Y.: Orbis Books, 1976), 204. Pope John XXIII, *Mater et Magistra,* May 15, 1961, #196–99, in Gremillion, *The Gospel of Peace and Justice,* 185–86. Pope John Paul II, *Laborem Exercens,* September 14, 1981, #19 (Rome: Vatican Polyglot Press), 67–72. Pope John Paul II, *Familiaris Consortio*, November 22, 1981, #46 (Boston: Pauline Books and Media, 1981), 71–73. For a systematic treatment of the right to procreate in the social encyclicals, David Hollenbach, "The Right to Procreate and its Social Limitation: A Systematic Study of Value Conflict in Roman Catholic Ethics" (Ph.D. dissertation, Yale University, 1975).

53 Martha Nussbaum, *Sex and Social Justice* (New York: Oxford, 1999), 50.

54 There is serious disagreement, of course, on the question of when the full panoply of rights would apply to offspring—at conception or at some later point in development. The moral status of the fetus is far too complex a question to take up in this space and I intentionally set it aside here. Since the sort of reproductive decisions about which one might want to draw limits are, at this point in the discussion, those involving practices like cloning or genetic engineering for specific characteristics, I have in mind reproductive choices about offspring one intends to bring to term.

55 For background on the Vatican's engagement with the population issue, see my "Reflections on Population Policy from the Roman Catholic Tradition," in *Beyond the Numbers*, edited by Laurie Mazur (Washington, D.C.: Island Press, 1994), 330–40.

56 See Pius XII, "Fundamental Laws Governing Conjugal Relations," (October 29, 1951), in *Medical Ethics: Sources of Catholic Teachings,* edited by Kevin D. O'Rourke and Philip Boyle, 2d edition (Washington, D.C.: Georgetown University Press, 1995), 207–08.

57 This is most clearly articulated in the Vatican "Instruction on Respect for Human Life in Its Origin and on the Dignity of Procreation (*Donum Vitae*)" (Congregation for the Doctrine of the Faith, March 19, 1987), #1, in *Gift of Life: Catholic Scholars Respond to the Vatican Instruction,* edited by Edmund D. Pellegrino, John Collins Harvey, and John P. Langan (Washington, D.C.: Georgetown University Press, 1990), pp. 4, 30. This same document also addresses the extent of the right; it is "not the right to have a child, but only the right to perform those natural acts which are per se ordered to procreation" (#8). See also "Perspectives on Population Policy," address by Bishop Jan Schotte to the U.N. International Conference

on Population, (August 8, 1984), reprinted in *Origins* 14, no. 133 (1984): 205–08.

58 Pope Paul VI, *Octogesima Adveniens* (May 14, 1971), #13, in Gremillion, *The Gospel of Peace and Justice*, 491.

59 John Paul II, *Familiaris Consortio* (1981), #23, in *Origins* 11, no. 28–29 (December 24, 1981): 438–66.

60 For a critical analysis of the family in Roman Catholic social thought, see Margaret A. Farley, "The Church and the Family: An Ethical Task," *Horizons,* 10, no. 1 (1983): 50–71. See also Hollenbach, "The Right to Procreate and its Social Limitations: A Systematic Study of Value Conflict in Roman Catholic Ethics."

61 See, e.g., Christine Gudorf, *Body, Sex and Pleasure: Reconstructing Christian Sexual Ethics* (Cleveland, Ohio: Pilgrim Press, 1994); Andre Guindon, *The Sexual Language: An Essay in Moral Theology* (Toronto: University of Ottowa Press, 1976); James B. Nelson, *Embodiment: An Approach to Sexuality and Christian Theology* (Minneapolis: Augsburg Publishing House, 1978).

62 *Pacem in Terris*, #53, in Gremillion, *The Gospel of Peace and Justice,* 213.

CHAPTER FIVE

ASSISTED REPRODUCTION AND ACCESS TO HEALTH CARE

> *A full account of health must allow for forms of personal and social life in which those made vulnerable by incurable disease, permanent disability, or immanent death remain full members of our human community, with opportunities to continue exercising their personal freedom.*

> —Alastair V. Campbell, *Health as Liberation: Medicine, Theology and the Quest for Justice*

Among the many human rights mentioned in *Pacem in Terris's* ambitious table is the right to medical care.[1] As in the case of other social, economic, and political rights defended by John XXIII, the right to medical care is a way of spelling out the meaning of respect for human dignity. To acknowledge the fundamental equality of all persons is to recognize both their equal potential for human flourishing and their equal vulnerability before the threat of illness, disability, and death. Access to health care is important in a just society for the same reason that access to a range of political and economic goods is important. Rights, understood in this way, protect the necessary conditions for social participation, self-determination, and the pursuit of opportunity.

But it has not been easy to define the content of a "right to health care" in the United States, let alone to reach consensus on the force of such an idea for public policy. The Clinton plan was an attempt, if not to assert a fundamental right to a "decent minimum" level of health care, at least to articulate the duties of government to assure basic equity in access to the medical goods its citizens need and value. It failed, in part because it fell victim to powerful counter-interests, but in part because there is a long tradition in the United States of treating health care as, at the same time, a commodity, an entitlement, and a dispensation of charity. Both the managed care revolution that followed and its backlash illustrate the ambiguous status of medical goods.

122

While managed care may have brought into relief the business dimensions of the physician-patient relationship that have always been there, many people are profoundly uncomfortable, even outraged, to find themselves "medical consumers" at the mercy of the market.

This chapter presses further the implications of the account of health and the goals of medicine developed earlier. What follows from thinking about health not just in terms of particular individuals, but also in terms of individuals as family members, workers, members of the community, and political beings? How would we understand the meaning and scope of a right to health care if we thought of it as a shared or common good and as having to do with the conditions for full participation in the human community? What are the consequences for our approach to the questions of distributive justice in health care if, as Cassell suggests, we measure medicine's success not merely by survival or length of life but by function and the ability of persons to pursue important personal and social goals? And what is the place of assisted reproduction in such a medicine?

The interpretation of the scope of social obligations to guarantee access to health care that follows is indebted to Catholic social teaching. The conclusions I draw, therefore, are dependent in obvious ways on theological presuppositions about, for example, the nature of the self, the meaning of human dignity, and the force of special claims by the most marginalized. Such a theological foundation, however, need not render the analysis that follows invalid for questions of policy in our current pluralistic context. Grounded in a natural law ethic, the Catholic social tradition presumes a moral realism and a form of moral knowledge that is independent of revelation. Although it is not assumed that believers and nonbelievers will share at all times the same conclusions or exhibit the same moral motivations, it is assumed that dialogue on moral issues is possible and that ethical language is accessible across traditions. Charles Dougherty's *Back to Reform* is a good example of an argument for health care reform that is addressed to a broad audience, but that employs many of the central themes that characterize Catholic social teaching, for example, the priority of the common good, human dignity as the foundation of society, and the interconnection of rights and responsibilities.[2] His understanding of the content of human dignity and the nature of a just society is obviously influenced by the Catholic tradition; however, the appeals he makes for equitable access to a basic level of health care do not rest on theological convictions.

Martha Nussbaum has also demonstrated that it is possible to draw universal conclusions about human flourishing and thus about what is needed for a life that is "truly human" that do not require consensus on the level of metaphysics. The capabilities account that she has developed with Amartya Sen judges political arrangements by the question: "How well have the people of [this] country been enabled to perform the central human functions?" The table of human functional capabilities that she invokes—for example, being able to live a life of normal length, to have good health, to move freely from place to place, to enjoy sexual satisfaction and choice in matters of reproduction, to use the senses, to have attachments to things and persons outside oneself, to engage in practical reasoning, and to be able to live with concern for others and for the physical world—is based on an experiential and historical universalism. Surely across time and culture, she argues, we find commonalities of need and aspiration. We do not need to adopt an essentialist anthropology to see that human beings are creatures "such that, provided with the right educational and material support, they can become fully capable of the major human functions," or, therefore, to agree that those capabilities exert a moral claim on every human society.[3] Nussbaum's presuppositions about the normative character of human dignity and her conclusion that "moving all citizens above a basic threshold of capability should be taken as a central social goal" have much in common with the social and political vision of the Catholic tradition. Nussbaum's is a pointedly liberal argument. Clearly there will be important differences between her version of social justice and what we find in the encyclical tradition, just as there are important differences between her account of basic human capabilities and the account a theologian might give. As Lisa Sowle Cahill points out, for example, Nussbaum gives very little weight to kinship as part of human flourishing and, as a result, little attention to what might be necessary to support and sustain family life. Still, Nussbaum shows that it is not futile to suggest that a rich and full version of human flourishing can be used to judge the equity of social arrangements, even in circumstances where there are multiple and competing understandings of the Good.

To say that we can use language like "human flourishing" or "the common good" fruitfully in debate over access to medical care does not mean that we can move easily and without tension from analysis of the sort that will be offered here to public policy. There are both practical and theoretical limits to the force of ultimately theological convictions in shaping law and practice. It is probably impossible and even imprudent to try to ban donor methods of assisted reproduction on the basis of the theological objections earlier expressed. In the same way, it is unlikely that a bias for the poor strong enough to override the economic opportunism that pervades managed care can be cultivated in a highly individualistic society such as ours. The point is only that efforts to ask what level of access to basic goods ought to be guaranteed in a just society need not founder hopelessly on the acknowledgment of pluralism. Moreover, although the question of how theological convictions might inform public debate over access to health care is important, what follows is primarily a theological exercise. It is possible to proceed, at least at this point, unconstrained by the practical and political considerations that would necessarily enter in were we developing a full-blown policy position. That said, let us turn to the problem of defining the scope of a "right to health care."

Human Dignity and Access to Health Care

Earlier we described rights as "shares in the basic conditions of human well-being," "reciprocal accountabilities that are binding for all persons." Under this description, a right to health care is a share in what is needed to promote and protect the basic physical and psychological dimensions of well-being. John XXIII includes the guarantee of access to health care among the obligations of a just or humane society because health is a universal necessity for the "proper development of life." In a sense, then, an argument for a right to health care in the Catholic social tradition follows from the same sort of question Nussbaum asks: "How are the people of [this] community to be enabled to perform the central human functions?" In a theological perspective, the spiritual dimensions of well-being are as important as the physical and social. Thus, in places the theologian is likely to define somewhat differently those "central functions" or capabilities that ought to be the subject of social justice. She will hold protection against the threat of debilitating illness to be a value, for example, not only because it is a precondition for realizing social projects and personal goals, but because it is a precondition (albeit not a necessary one) for pursuing the invitation of relationship with God. But what is at stake for John XXIII in insisting that social justice includes acknowledgment of what are often called positive rights—that is, to food, shelter, health care, education, job training, and so on—is what is at stake for Nussbaum: the creation of social conditions under which human capacities for self-determination, initiative, and meaningful contribution to the community can be exercised.

In a short treatise on health care rationing published in 1991, the Catholic Health Association (CHA) argued that "when the health care system becomes dysfunctional or people are denied access to basic care, government has a duty to act on the behalf of those people and for the good of society as a whole."[4] Two important presuppositions underlie this claim. First, it is presupposed that at least one of the tasks of government is to secure the good working of different social agents and bodies in the service of collective human welfare. The common good is achieved, CHA argues, "when communities of mutual concern and responsibility—in this case, health care providers, the insurance industry, government, and the public—work on behalf of all."[5] Second, it is presupposed that health care is a social or public good. Equitable access to health care is a matter for justice because illness threatens individual human dignity, but it is a matter for social justice because human dignity is secured only through social cooperation. Health care is a public rather than private good in part because science and medicine are maintained by social investments. But it is also public in the sense of being necessary for realizing the opportunities and obligations of the common good, such as governance, work and leisure, family life, and intellectual development.

What would follow from claiming a fundamental right to health care on these grounds? First, arguing for equitable access to health care on the basis of a common human dignity would seem clearly to favor egalitarian systems for allocating health care over libertarian or utilitarian. A libertarian theory of allocation holds that social arrangements should maximize individual liberty and, as far as possible, protect the freedom of individuals to acquire and enjoy personal property. It is reasonable to assume that a rational person would want protection from unanticipated health crises. Therefore, individuals should be free to protect themselves in whatever way they wish, such as by purchasing insurance or setting aside resources. Health care needs are not, however, clearly distinguishable from other interests and preferences; such needs are not, in this view, special in such a way as to place claims on society that would override individual liberty. Thus, while charity may dictate aiding those who do not have resources to deal with health crises, justice does not demand it.

Utilitarian theories of allocation take as their goal the maximization of overall utility or "preference satisfaction,"—that is, the greatest good for the greatest number. It is possible to derive a right to health care from utilitarian social theory on the grounds that social welfare is best served when members of the society are protected from serious harms such as illness and premature death. But utilitarian models of allocation differ from egalitarian in that they allow for trade-offs and partial allocations as required by an overall concern for the balance between public and private benefit, and may introduce factors such as merit and projected social contribution into the specification of health care rights.

In contrast, egalitarian theories of distributive justice presuppose the essential equality of all persons and, by extension, equality in both need and opportunity. If each person's welfare is to count equally, then disparities in access to basic or essential goods or opportunities are unjust and should be remedied. Since all are vulnerable to health care crises, all should receive equal consideration in allocation decisions.

The second thing that follows from Catholic social teaching's account of the common good is a particular view of the role of the state in guaranteeing collective welfare. Government need not provide health care services as such, but is responsible, rather, for assuring that whatever mechanisms are adopted for distributing health care (or any other basic good) are just and for securing a floor of well-being when the activity of the institutions concerned fails to do so. Private enterprise, therefore, is not incompatible with this kind of egalitarianism. However, if the market fails to generate or distribute goods to meet the essential needs of all, or even if does so without respect for human dignity, it is ultimately a failure of government.

A Decent Minimum

If we make access to health care a question of fundamental or shared human dignity, some principles for allocating goods will be more fitting than others. As Gene Outka argued in a now classic essay, to distribute health care according to the principle "to each according to the ability to pay," or "to each according to merit and/or social contribution" denies the equal susceptibility of persons—good and evil, prudent and foolish—both to illness and its often catastrophic effects. If we are equal in our essential embodied needs and equally vulnerable to death and disability, the only fitting principles for deciding who deserves to be treated are "to each according to need," or "similar treatment for similar cases."[6]

But even if we agree that "need" or "dignity" is the appropriate basis for the allocation of health care as a social good, we still have the problem of priorities: Which health needs are essential? When is the denial of a particular treatment a violation of human dignity even if no one is to get it? "Need" or "benefit" are necessary features of any claim to health care. But, as we previously observed, they are far from sufficient for defining the scope of legitimate claims for health care. For one thing, no society can afford to guarantee that all its members have access to the medical care they "need" or from which they will benefit. Unless a society has unlimited resources or pursues health as its only social good, it would be irrational for it to adopt such a goal.[7] Moreover, as we saw earlier in our discussion of the status of assisted reproduction, it is nearly impossible to distinguish neatly between "needs" and "wants" in the context of health care. Except when we are ill, health is not even a good in itself. It is a precondition for pursuing whatever ends we value and one standard among others for assessing the quality of our lives.

The right to health care is usually interpreted as a right to a "decent minimum." For most people, this means something like access to primary and preventive care, prenatal and well-baby care, necessary hospitalization, mental health and substance abuse services, specialty care when called for and, perhaps, prescription drugs. Determining what should constitute a "decent minimum" is, of course, notoriously difficult. It is in part a matter of economics, that is, how much a particular nation can afford to spend on health care given other needs and investments. It is also, in part, a matter of medicine: What treatments are most effective in a given set of circumstances or what treatments should be considered the standard of care?[8] Given that economic status in any area fluctuates and medicine evolves, consensus concerning the content of a decent minimum will be inevitably both local and provisional. In addition,

already existing material conditions will shape perceptions about what falls
above or below the minimum.

Still, adopting the criterion that "everyone is to receive an 'adequate' or
'decent minimum' level of care" avoids the most serious problems entailed in
commitments to meet every individual's health care needs.[9] Here it is acknowledged that there will be some services excluded that might be legitimately needed or from which patients might derive benefit, even great benefit.
It is also possible that there could be aggregate inequalities in the level of
health care received across the society. As long as a floor of "adequate benefits" exists to which everyone has access, it is not a failure of distributive justice if an upper tier of services exists to which those with means also have
access. Moreover, as Allen Buchanan argues, the criterion of an "adequate" or
"decent" minimum "allows us to adjust the level of services to be provided as
a matter of right to relevant social circumstances and also allows for the possibility that as a society becomes more affluent the floor provided by the decent minimum should be raised."[10]

How useful the argument for a "right to a decent minimum" is for defining the obligations of a just society depends, however, on the content of "decent minimum." If "decent minimum" is defined, as it sometimes is, simply in
terms of "basic needs," or "most essential health care needs," it is not obvious
that we have advanced much beyond "to each according to need." Especially
when we are reasoning in terms of what types of care we ourselves are likely
to need, the table of "essentials" can be almost hopelessly expansive. Philip
Keane argues that, from the standpoint of Catholic social teaching, we can ascertain the meaning of a "decent minimum" in the same way as we ascertain
the meaning of a "living wage": If all persons can live in reasonable and frugal comfort, their true needs (as opposed to wants) are being met and justice
is achieved.[11] This way of framing the obligation has obvious appeal. But "reasonable and frugal comfort" is a relative judgment, dependent on existing levels of expectation that, in some cases, might already be too high. In addition,
in the context of health care, what is needed to bring everyone to a perceived
level of "reasonable and frugal comfort," might, under some circumstances,
simply exceed social resources.

To begin to set priorities for a health care system and, ultimately, to examine the place of assisted reproductive technologies within those priorities, we
need to look at the function of health care, to ask what health care is *for* and why
investments are important, not just for individuals, but for societies. Earlier, we
drew from the International Goals of Medicine Project a description of health as
the "absence of significant malady; the ability to pursue one's vital goals; and
the ability to function in ordinary social and work contexts."[12] To describe health
this way is compatible with understanding access to health care as a "share in
the basic conditions of well-being," in what is necessary for social agency. It is
also compatible with understanding the rationale for social investments as ori-

ented toward human flourishing, toward the development and maintenance of a certain set of important and shared human capabilities. If we begin with this description of health, we can narrow the normative and programmatic question to this: What level of health care is needed to guarantee, as much as possible, the "absence of significant malady, the ability to pursue one's vital goals, and the ability to function in ordinary social and work contexts"? What is needed, in other words, to allow each member of society, according to his or her own capacities, to live—paraphrasing Callahan—a "good, mortal life"?

Sufficiency

We acknowledged earlier that judgments about what constitutes a "good, mortal life," just as judgments about what constitutes a "significant malady," one's "vital goals," and "ordinary social and work contexts" are necessarily local and dialogical. To be sure, as Nussbaum argues, there are some human potentialities, some functions that "are so central that they seem definitive of a life that is truly human."[13] To be able to live to the end of one's normal life span or to be free of the sort of affliction that makes any meaningful engagement with others or the world impossible would count as necessary for a "good mortal life" under any circumstances. But what is needed for a minimum level of function or participation in ordinary social and work contexts might differ dramatically across cultures and across economic systems. Therefore, on this level, it is possible only to suggest broad principles for determining an adequate level of social investments or guarantees. But even broad principles are helpful in beginning to make the link between the conditions for social agency and the importance of health care.

In *What Kind of Life,* Callahan lays out a framework for setting societal priorities in health care.[14] It is worth considering as a way of thinking concretely about what health care would look like in a society that adopted such a view of the goals of medicine and ultimately for thinking about the pursuit of parenthood within it.

Callahan's strategy rests on several of the assumptions we have made concerning the rationale for social investments in health and health care:

1. good health is to be pursued in order to enhance individual flourishing and the overall welfare of society; health is a means to important ends, but not an end in itself;
2. aging, sickness, and death are intrinsic to the human condition; a prudent society places limits on its aspirations and expenditures for life extension and the cure of disease in all its forms;
3. a society has a sufficient level of health when "its citizens are on the whole healthy enough to pursue its common purposes and participate in

the life of its private communities, and when poor health is in general no longer an impediment to the functioning of its major social and political institutions."[15]

Defining health as concerned with the living of a "good, mortal life" yields a bias for investments in life-enhancing over merely life-prolonging treatments, population health over a generalized assault on disease, and basic primary and emergency care over curative therapies that serve the individual needs of a small number of people at great cost. A just and sensible system, Callahan argues, is one that strikes a balance between caring and curing, with priority given to those who are presently most marginalized; it is a system that guarantees a minimal level of adequate care for all, but that is prepared to set whatever upper limits to the pursuit of benefits for individuals are necessary to assure adequate care for all.

A "minimum level of adequate care" for Callahan includes: full support for *caring*—that is, support for the sick, disabled, and dying to reconnect them, as much as possible, to the life of the community; investment in public health measures that promote "general societal health," as well as access to primary and emergency care; and access to "more individualized forms of care" compatible with prudent overall societal investments in health care.[16] How do we determine when "more individualized forms of care" are compatible with "prudent overall societal investments in health care"? Callahan suggests the following standards for establishing the burden of proof in a reasonable public debate: (1) promise of serving public interest (for example, meeting age-group needs, redressing socioeconomic inequities, and reducing infectious potential); (2) promise of relieving long-term care demand (for example, reducing public and private burden of care for the aged or disabled, promoting independence in living); (3) promise of meeting basic human needs, physical, psychological, and functional; and (4) cost-effectiveness, judged both in terms of expense and medical, social, and cultural benefit.[17]

The strength of Callahan's proposal is in its appreciation for the place of individual needs or claims within an overall orientation toward the common good and its recognition of the inescapably social or political character of the exercise of setting systemic priorities. It shares certain of the values central to the Catholic social tradition: the interdependence of rights and responsibilities; the importance of attending to the role of social decisions in constructing the conditions of possibility for human flourishing, individually and collectively; and the prima facie priority given to the most marginalized. Callahan's insistence on the importance of caring for the chronically and terminally ill fills out the account we have given of health as a capacity for agency. Reconnecting those whose diminished capacities alienate them from the community is as valuable as protecting and developing those capacities in the well.

Moreover, it is assumed that the burdens of rationing care should be distributed equitably with an eye to the impact of allocation decisions on communities as well as on individuals, and with an eye to the qualitative as well as quantitative dimensions of the effectiveness of care. Callahan takes for granted that the work of determining sufficiency, and whatever will lie beyond, is a process of negotiation, which requires the participation of those who will be affected most directly by the decisions but which is not simply a "winner take all" contest between contesting parties. Most important, in arguing for a reorientation of medical priorities away from the all-out defeat of death and disease, he constructs a way of thinking about systemic priorities that taps the broad resources of the community. Death is not only a limit condition on the aspirations of medicine; it is a personal journey that can be profoundly marginalizing. The obligation to care aggressively continues even when the battle for a cure appropriately ceases. When our most fundamental concern becomes caring well for those who are, as he puts it, "already existing, but poorly," we open up possibilities for thinking beyond medical services when we talk about the priority of care.

To be sure, there are problems with this framework for systemic reform. For one thing, it requires a crucial conceptual shift in thinking about the allocation of health care from an individual matrix to a social matrix, a shift that has proven nearly impossible to effect in the United States. One of the many reasons that the Clinton plan failed was our long-standing cultural resistance to setting aside vital self-interest in the pursuit of social goals. Another reason was that its support for regional oversight boards implied recognition of the need for global rationing strategies. The late Richard McCormick often observed that we Americans seem to accept rationing only when we believe that we are in a state of emergency. At least in 1994, those who had health insurance did not find the status quo all that objectionable and certainly did not see either the rising costs of health care or the growing numbers of un- and underinsured Americans as a "crisis." A third and related problem is the difficulty of accepting limitations in care as we move from the statistical patient to the real or identified patient. It is one thing to agree, for example, that aggressive treatment for very premature infants should not be a priority; it is another thing to accept the judgment that *your* very premature infant will not receive aggressive care. It is one thing to argue that we should be willing to give up our often obsessive and frantic assault on death and aging. It is another to contemplate letting go as one approaches one's own dying or the diminishment of age. The sharpest criticism of Callahan's vision for health reform has concerned the perceived implications of arguing for a medicine oriented toward facilitating a "reasonable life span" for the care of particular aging patients.

An additional problem is that of coordinating the quality of care on various levels. If a health care system allows for two or three tiers, as Callahan's ideal would, if it allows for a buyout or "buymore" option on the level of individual curative therapies, there is always the challenge of maintaining a sufficient quality of care at the level of "adequacy" or the "decent minimum." It is also possible that the availability of goods or services on the upper tiers will drive up expectations regarding sufficiency on the lowest tier.

These are important issues, but we do not have to resolve all of them in order to profit from Callahan's attempt to lay out the implications of treating the pursuit of health as a question both of individual human flourishing and social welfare. Neither do we have to be able to predict exactly how this conceptual framework would be applied, since, as we argued above, application assumes a specific political process. The argument for systemic reform above is brief, broad, and necessarily general. What Callahan gives us, however, is an important moral orientation, a set of values—sufficiency, sustainability, equity, and interdependence—for weighing the importance of social investments in medicine. In addition, he gives us a way of talking about the priority of different sorts of health-related needs and interests within an overarching commitment to the common good. With this in mind, let us turn to the question of assisted reproduction and its place in arguments for the "right to a decent minimum."

Investments in Reproducing

In the course of this book we have made several important claims about infertility and assisted reproduction that would be useful at this stage to recall. Early on, we called into question the false distinction between IVF and other forms of treatment in debates over reimbursements for infertility. The effort to jettison the question of how far society ought to go to facilitate genetic parenthood by simply excluding expensive and sophisticated therapies is, we argued, both illusory and dangerous. The fact is that a social price is being paid for infertility, without responsible reflection on the nature of those investments. We also called into question the assumption that infertility can be neatly distinguished from other conditions or maladies for which we assume medical responses are appropriate. Rather, if we agree with the characterization of health as a capacity for acting in the world, for pursuing vital goals, it is difficult to see how we would not include infertility among medicine's legitimate goals. Biological reproduction is not only a prima facie "vital goal" for individuals, but it is a basic dimension of our common interpretations of human flourishing. The important question is how far ought medicine go to assist infertile individuals and at what price?

We also resisted the tendency to treat questions of reproduction as wholly private matters. As a practical matter, choices about assisted reproduction involve social costs and social consequences that belie arguments for privacy. It is not only possible to think of reproduction and assisted reproduction in the context of the common good, but necessary to do so, even to propose moral limits on the choices any individual might make in reproduction.

We have made claims about the shape of an "equitable and sustainable" health care system as well. If it makes sense to think of health in terms of social agency or function and in terms of social connection, then the question to be posed to any system is whether or not the type and level of care needed to pursue common purposes and enjoy a minimum level of participation in the life of the community is guaranteed to all. With Callahan, we argued that it is legitimate—and from the perspective of the option for the poor, morally enjoined—to set upper limits to the guarantee of benefits to individuals when limits are necessary to assure adequate care for all.

In light of these claims, what can we conclude about the status of assisted reproduction? To the extent that we are concerned in the delivery of health care with the way in which illness and impairment separate human beings from valued relationships, goals, and events, we should be concerned with the care of the infertile. If we are to take the experience of infertility seriously, then we need to see it as an assault on the integrity of the self, a body-failure that shares the features of illness in general. However, placing questions of access to treatment for infertility in the context of the common good means that we cannot see infertility merely as an experience of *individual selves*. From the perspective of the common good, the question of whether infertile persons ought to be assisted in reproduction becomes more than a matter of whether the therapy available is efficacious or the therapeutic approach chosen appropriate. To be weighed in the balance are the implications of expenditures on infertility for meeting the needs of the poor and the near-poor for life-sustaining goods and services; the effect of therapeutic responses to infertility on the social conditions of reproduction; and the significance of this particular form of compromised social participation vis-à-vis the forms experienced by others in one's society. To defend the rights of the most marginalized to the minimum conditions for participation in the common life we will also have to assess procreative technologies in the context of existing imbalances in social power relations. If we agree with Beverly Harrison that "no one has a right to [the satisfaction of] luxury or even to less essential 'enhancement' needs . . . at the price of another's basic dignity or physical survival," and that no one has a right to liberty that is "sustained by dehumanizing structures of exploitation," the costs to be counted in an analysis also include the impact of procreative technologies on efforts to achieve racial, economic, and gender equality.[18] The right to seek advanced infertility services or to be assisted in pursuing treatment will not be defensible if it can only be honored at the expense of the survival needs of some individuals or groups, or by maintaining an order of privilege that advantages some individuals and groups by disadvantaging others.

What follows is a "modest" or "cautious" argument for a right to assisted reproduction, one that calls into question the current practice of discriminating between the rich infertile and the poor infertile with respect to treatment, but one that places the issue within the larger questions of social justice raised above and, therefore, defends limitations on what might be said to be owed to infertile individuals.

Equity and Access

If advanced infertility treatment is defensible as a medical good on the basis that it addresses impairments to a primary human function that is related to human dignity, flourishing, and participation in the common life, it ought to be available on an equitable basis. As we argued earlier, to leave access to infertility treatment as a matter of the free market privatizes infertility and fails to attend sufficiently to the reality of race and class bias in the distribution of this arguably important resource. In addition, it trivializes the importance of access to care, especially in the lives of women. For most people, reproduction is one of the reasons why well-being matters, and why rights to life, a decent wage, shelter, or medical care are so important. Bearing and rearing children is a reasonable feature of a rational life plan and a part of the meaning of human flourishing. It is fair to argue that the conditions of possibility for choosing reproduction should be included in the functional needs a just and adequate medicine should protect.

But the procreative interests of infertile persons have to be evaluated in light of the obligation of society to provide universal access to a decent minimum level of care. From our reading of Catholic social teaching, we saw that securing the fundamental well-being of the marginalized has priority over the interests of the well-off, and guaranteeing basic primary and emergency care takes precedence over curative therapies that benefit a small number of individuals. It can be argued, therefore, that the moral claim of those lacking access to basic health care supersedes the freedom of others to pursue less essential care. Infertility compromises flourishing, but it does not by itself foreclose basic opportunity. Infertility treatment serves as much an "enhancement" as an essential need, as childbearing presupposes satisfaction of essential needs. While the state of involuntary childlessness can color all other life experiences, it does not present the same obstacles as other impairments with respect to an individual's ability to learn or to work, to provide shelter, and to otherwise take care of essential needs, or to engage in relationships. While providing access to treatment for infertility is a reasonable goal within a health care system, it is not defensible at the price of basic or "decently minimum" care for those not being now served.

The goal of providing universal access to basic primary and preventative care is not necessarily or ultimately in conflict with the goal of providing equitable access to the means for addressing reproductive impairments.

For one thing, access to routine and responsive gynecological care; sex education, including education about the prevention of disease and the natural scope of fertility; safe and effective contraception; and sufficient social and economic support for women in the care of children so that career-seeking women are not regularly forced to delay childbearing would, in the long run, do more to assure broad reproductive health than appropriating funds to treat infertility when it appears. Although a focus on preventative care or social restructuring will never eliminate entirely the need for the kind of restorative and compensatory treatment now being offered, a more focused attention on good basic care for women shows promise of naturally reducing the need for such treatment.

Even where access to care means access to infertility treatment, the needs of the infertile in the United States are not necessarily in mortal conflict with the needs of the uninsured or underinsured for basic services, although they are often portrayed that way. As we argued earlier, the cost of adding infertility services to a basic benefits package, even with a guarantee of two attempts at IVF, would not have the devastating impact on global health costs as we usually assume.[19] There are, of course, many places in the world where the difficulty of providing for the most essential needs of the population would render the goal of providing access to costly infertility treatment indefensible even if there are reasons for defending the treatment in itself. In parts of the developing world, where poverty is deep and relentless, the effect of diseases like AIDS devastating, and expenditures on health care a fraction of what they are in the United States, arguing for guaranteed access to infertility treatment seems pointless, even though the childless woman in those same parts of the world may suffer much more devastating social stigma than her North American counterpart. But the failure of the United States to guarantee access to basic health care to all of its citizens is not fundamentally a problem of impossibility but of will. In this context, there are conflicts between the interests of the infertile and the needs/interests of those without access to basic health care, but they are related to deeper systemic problems that are, in principle, correctable.

Whatever shape the debate over universal access takes, however, it is safe to assume that it will be impossible simply to extend access to infertility treatment to everyone who would like to use it for whatever purpose, or even to offer unlimited services to everyone who is involuntarily childless in the United States. So what strategies might be adopted for suggesting whose needs (or what kinds of needs) would be addressed as guaranteed benefits, if at least some are to be? How, in other words, might we begin to decide what forms of assisted reproduction, as curative therapies, meet the principles we defended above?

First, if a general move is made from treating advanced infertility services as a market commodity, which is necessary for all the reasons discussed earlier, to treating it as a health care good, the problem of agreeing on a definition of infertility is inescapable. In current practice, the frustration of any desire for biological parenthood is called "infertility." Given our understanding of health as the "absence of significant malady, the ability to pursue one's vital goals and the ability to function in ordinary social and work contexts," as well as the argument we have offered for the appropriate goals of medicine, it makes sense to narrow the concept of infertility to indicate a condition following from a "reproductive impairment." Infertility, for the purposes of this argument, is an impairment giving rise to a normative claim insofar as it is the frustration of a physical capacity that results in the inability to act in the world in an important way, that is, through procreation.

If we use infertility by reason of "reproductive impairment" as the broad criterion for access, some forms of involuntary childlessness now treated by artificial reproduction would not qualify. Other forms that are now routinely excluded would be included. Single women or men, or gay or lesbian couples, for example, who seek donor-assisted reproduction would not have a strong claim to guaranteed access, nor would individuals who turn to reproductive technology for convenience or for purposes of maximizing control over the outcome. The unmarried woman or man who desires to reproduce sexually but cannot because of a blocked fallopian tube or poor sperm motility would have a claim. The single woman who wants children but lacks a male partner and the single woman who wants children but suffers from a tubal obstruction both experience involuntary childlessness; only the latter case, however, exhibits what could be called a "body-based" frustration of potentiality.

Distinguishing rights to access this way could appear to play into the hands of those who might wish to allocate services based on prevailing sexual norms. But what is at issue is not what makes a person a fit parent, but what is a legitimate claim on the health care system. If the overall goal of health care is the capacity to live a good, mortal life and the proximate goal is to guarantee a basic level of participation in the life of the community, it makes sense to isolate health care claims according to their relation to some account of "normal species functioning," or "normal opportunity range" or the "human potential ordinarily open to an individual at any particular stage in life."[20] Some rough principle like normal opportunity range is at work anytime we try to distinguish the needs properly attended to by medicine from other limitations and obstacles to happiness. It is what we assume when we differentiate, for example, between the "need" for a leg-lengthening procedure in order to be tall enough to play professional basketball and the "need" for a kidney transplant. Having functioning kidneys is a part of "normal species function" in a way that being seven feet tall is not.

A standard such as "normal opportunity" is admittedly crude and not altogether satisfying. What we take to be "normal species functioning" is to some extent socially constructed and overlaid with cultural notions of "health," "beauty, and "normality." As such, it is a vulnerable standard, open to manipulation by powerful social, political, and economic forces and subject to change as understandings of the "normal" change. This standard may prove even more vulnerable as we move fully into the genetic age, in which accepted physical limits and metaphysical boundaries are falling to the new possibilities opened up by new technologies. Yet, if for the sake of weighing social investments in health care, we accept a view of health as a means rather than an end in itself, as an important but not self-exhaustive dimension of human flourishing, it is necessary to work from an account of what might reasonably be expected of the human body in the pursuit of that good, mortal life. To say that we ought to be concerned with addressing infertility as an aspect of normal species functioning is another way of saying that we should be concerned with the role of medical care in helping people pursue their vital goals or function in ordinary work and social contexts. Not all forms of involuntary childlessness follow from a body-based frustration of normal reproductive potential, but some clearly do and that is the class of claims with which we are concerned here.

We have to acknowledge as well that the complexity of infertility as a phenomenon makes the effort to isolate the meaning of "reproductive impairment" inescapably difficult. For one thing, infertility is characterized more by the frustration of a potentiality than by the loss of a function. Therefore, it can be difficult to determine onset and sometimes impossible to explain. A problem in conceiving often becomes clinical infertility at the point where a patient insists on more specialized treatment. A premature diagnosis of infertility might mean the premature receipt of expensive and unnecessary treatment; a delayed diagnosis might cost a patient his or her window of opportunity for a successful outcome.

Also complicating matters is the fact that infertility arises in a *collaborative matrix*. Sexual reproduction is a two-party event, where a successful outcome is dependent on factors relative to each party and also to their interaction. It is possible, therefore, to become infertile by virtue of one's choice of partner. It would be useful to be able to sharpen the definition of "reproductive impairment" so that it applied in all cases to a condition existing in a particular individual. However, the lines are simply not as neat here as they are with regard to other impairments. A husband's inability to walk affects a couple and a family, but the impairment can be located in one individual. This is just not so with forms of infertility. In clinical practice, a diagnosis of infertility is usually made when a couple has been unable to conceive following a year of unprotected intercourse or after six months of timed intercourse in cases in which the woman is in her mid-thirties or older or there is some reason to suspect impaired fertility in the couple. This seems a fair way of identifying a pool of candidates for further investigation or treatment, even though we are relying here again on a somewhat crude and imprecise standard.

Without pretending more precision than is possible, we are arguing here that the notion of "reproductive impairment" is a useful one for guiding broad allocation decisions. It is also useful for directing the goals and priorities of reproductive medicine. In attempting to isolate what kinds of involuntary childlessness might generate claims to access, we cannot escape also asking something about what the aims of reproductive medicine should be. We have seen that infertility is a complex crisis, with physical, psychosexual, social, and existential features. Reproductive technologies cannot address many of the dimensions of suffering for the infertile. They cannot solve a spiritual crisis, for example, or repair a marriage that has splintered under the strain of disappointment. What technology can hope to do is restore function or compensate for impaired function.

An emphasis on infertility as a body-based frustration of a natural and valuable potentiality yields two biases in the assessment of reproductive services: (1) a bias toward the restoration or enhancement of function over the replacement of function; (2) a bias toward integrated or holistic approaches to the treatment of infertility. Given that the motivation for addressing infertility comes, in this analysis, from concerns for well-being and the recognition of the significance of reproduction as a dimension of human agency, we should be as concerned with the effort to restore reproductive capacity as with the ability to place it under ever greater clinical control. Whether it is more appropriate (safer, more effective, cheaper, etc.) in a given case to try to repair a damaged fallopian tube or to go directly to IVF is best left to clinical judgment. A bias for restoration gives us no hard and fast guideline for weighing investments in available therapies. However, efforts to explore pharmacological, immunological, and epidemiological approaches to female and male infertility, or to expand the possibilities for laser surgery in the control and treatment of endometriosis or refine the use of tuboplasty in the repair of fallopian tubes ought not to be abandoned in favor of finding ever better ways to bypass the reproductive system. In other words, we should question the present tendencies in reproductive medicine toward "producing children" versus enabling reproduction.

In addition, although a medical model is being proposed for distinguishing stronger from weaker claims on societal resources, a medical approach to infertility is far from adequate. The recognition that persons suffer more than one kind of crisis (not just physical, but emotional, spiritual, and social) because of involuntary childlessness implies a team approach to patient care, where emotional suffering is acknowledged with at least the same energy as physical impairment and where a range of approaches can be explored. Unlike some illness and impairments, infertility can be resolved equally well with or without medical intervention. Individuals should be helped from the beginning, therefore, to consider all the alternatives such as adoption, child-free living, and "low tech" or natural remedies as well as more advanced or medically sophisticated therapies. Self-help groups like those sponsored by Resolve have been helpful in this respect by bringing individuals together to learn how to cope, not only with the frustrations of trying to conceive, but with the deeper problem of involuntary childlessness. These groups are still, however, largely on the outskirts of the medical institutions, and referrals often come after a long period of unsuccessful treatment when the range of attractive alternatives has narrowed. Working though the adoption process can, in some cases, allow a couple to make a free and healthy choice to discontinue treatment that has become more burdensome than beneficial. However, institutional policies, which require individuals to state that they have ended infertility treatment before they can begin to explore adoption, sometimes keep the "adoption option" from really entering into the therapeutic process. In advocating for a holistic approach, therefore, we are also advocating attention to the construction of possibilities for addressing infertility.

At the Boundaries

We have argued thus far that ensuring access to treatment for infertility is consistent with commitments to creating social conditions for human flourishing and fostering certain forms of human agency. At least where involuntary childlessness follows from a body-failure or reproductive impairment, it is reasonable to argue that it ought to be considered alongside other important health care needs. Some of the most interesting questions for this framework pertain to what we might call "questionable reproductive impairments." Premature Ovarian Failure (POF) is an obvious candidate for treatment in this analysis. Setting aside for the moment the particular problems posed by the need for donor egg IVF in addressing POF, it makes sense to include patients who have experienced menopause before the statistical age of normal onset in the class of patients with normative reproductive impairments. But how should "natural" or age-appropriate menopause be considered here? Is age-appropriate menopause a "reproductive impairment?" How about secondary infertility resulting from voluntary sterilization?

If the concept of reproductive impairment is related to normal opportunity range for a particular stage in life, age-appropriate menopause is a rational criterion for exclusion. Despite the fact that it is difficult to define the onset of menopause in general terms, there is a well-documented decline in fertility as women move from their mid-thirties to their mid-forties. Citing dismal success rates, many fertility centers refuse to treat women who are older than 45, except in donor-egg programs.[21] Yet the very promise of therapies aimed at extending reproductive capacities is to render the concept of a "natural window of fertility" anachronistic. Some women will be free and able to care for children well only later in life. Why, one might argue, should we continue to identify the period of normal opportunity with the period of natural fertility?

Defending age limits on access to infertility treatment is controversial, although not inconsistent with the general approach taken here. The physical demands of pregnancy and childbirth and the ongoing physical, emotional, and social demands of childcare raise the question of whether declining fertility is a kind of "body wisdom" that ought to be respected. If we are concerned with fostering a health care system that acts on the assumption that aging, illness, and death are intrinsic dimensions of the human experience and need not be overcome at all costs, we should be concerned about attempts to extend fertility, such as banking frozen eggs for later use, which involve a denial of the reality of women's aging. Moreover, ensuring equitable access to the means for pursuing vital human goals includes, we have seen, a commitment to meeting age-group needs. It is reasonable to argue that overcoming reproductive impairments is a value for men and women within the age range for normal fertility, but equally reasonable to argue that there is no strong social obligation on either side of that range. Finally, the problem of delayed childbearing is at its roots a social problem and we should be wary of tendencies to gamely offer a medical solution. Rather than correcting, at great cost, the problem of impaired fertility in older women, we should be addressing the social and marital practices that place investments in career and investments in family at odds for so many women, encouraging choices to postpone motherhood. Not all interests in conceiving after menopause are the result of decisions to postpone childbearing, but to the extent that social conditions create forced choices, a commitment to the well-being of women demands attention to those conditions.

In most states where coverage for infertility is mandatory, secondary infertility after voluntary sterilization is excluded on the grounds that fertility has been intentionally impaired. This approach is compatible with an analysis of justice in health care that takes its bearings from a concern for the common good. Here it is assumed that individuals have some responsibility for maintaining their health and some accountability for the use of medical resources. The question of access in such cases could become less important with the introduction of apparently safe and effective long-term contraceptives. But at the present time reversing a decision for surgical sterilization can require expensive medical intervention. If the consequences of a decision to be sterilized are known and the process is undergone voluntarily, it is not unreasonable to argue that there exists no obligation to provide future assistance in pursuing procreation. Of course, individuals contemplating permanent sterilization are owed accurate information and an environment where a free choice about fertility is possible. Legitimate questions can be raised of the conditions under which decisions are made, especially by the poor. It is here, in asking those questions, that the obligations of social justice most appropriately come into play.

The availability of donor methods raises interesting questions that we earlier set aside. Let us return to them briefly before we conclude with the problem of determining internal limits to access. Recall that IVF and IVF-related therapies are often excluded as health care benefits on the grounds that they bypass rather than treat the condition of infertility. Earlier we argued that isolating these therapies on such grounds is unfair and inconsistent. It is important, however, to ask whether donor methods would admit to such criticism, given the argument for determining just access offered here. The question is whether treatment using donor gametes or a surrogate womb can be said to address infertility as a crisis of the self or whether it merely resolves the problem of involuntary childlessness within a relationship. A couple may give birth to a child who is genetically related to one partner, or perhaps to both if the donor is a gestational surrogate, but the infertile partner is said to be only a "vicarious reproducer." He or she can experience the joy of parenting but is in some sense or to some degree replaced by the donor with regard to reproductive agency. If the ability to successfully resolve the crisis of infertility has to do with receiving the assistance that enables one to conceive a child when it seemed impossible, or with accepting the "truth of one's being" when treatment fails, we can wonder if donor-assisted methods short-circuit the process by perpetuating denial.

Some early studies suggested that men whose partners underwent donor insemination had special difficulty resolving the self-esteem issues that accompany infertility. Some men, in addition, had a hard time establishing warm parental bonds with their AID children.[22] But the women who report conceiving with donor eggs do not, by and large, seem to have problems accepting donor IVF as a positive approach to infertility or bonding with the child or children produced.[23] If we can rely at all on the testimony of women who are members of Internet support groups dedicated to motherhood through egg donation, it seems that women come, very early in a donor-assisted pregnancy, to see their unborn child as fully "theirs" and the pregnancy as a work or expression of the self, even as they acknowledge the necessity of the donor's contribution and, in some cases, continue to long for a genetically related child. Given the intensely physical and intimate nature of pregnancy, it is not surprising that conceiving through a donor egg would hardly feel like "vicarious reproduction." Although it is difficult to know what weight to give anecdotal impressions of a relatively new practice such as egg donation, such impressions argue against a quick and easy dismissal of donor methods as simply bypassing infertility.

We earlier argued that donor methods of artificial insemination and IVF raise moral questions from the perspective of Christian and Catholic commitments to the unity of sexuality and reproduction. Although it would be difficult to bracket donor methods on such grounds in a public debate about the scope of guaranteed access to assisted reproduction, those are the considerations that would finally be most important in this analysis. The conclusion that donor methods cannot be justified even under a revised or "liberal" Catholic treatment of reproductive technologies cuts against fighting for their place as health care benefits even if they provide care we consider important. This would be an area in which concerns about the effect of a particular therapy on the social conditions for fully human reproduction would come into play, where concerns about the impact of technology would have weight as a matter of social justice even if the therapy as such met the general conditions of distributive justice accepted here.

In a discussion that has been more suggestive than exhaustive, we have tried to offer a prima facie case for defending equitable access to infertility treatment as a dimension of respect for human dignity. Infertility, as an obstacle to "normal opportunity," an impairment that impedes the pursuit of a vital human goal, is a matter of justice inasmuch as social justice demands the protection of conditions for basic human flourishing. We have attempted, at least in a general way, to suggest how we might distinguish between different claims to access, how we might weigh different sorts of involuntary childlessness, in determining what is fair treatment. Although we have explored the "who?" and the "what?" we have not yet faced the most pressing question: "How much?" Let us turn finally to it now.

Setting Limits

If equitable access is to be sought for those with the kind of reproductive impairments we have described—consistent, of course, with the obligation to meet basic needs—how far would a just society be expected to go in helping to overcome those impairments? The problem of defining limits is crucial if our aspirations for a health care system that is both equitable and sustainable have any hope of being realized. More important, the problem of limits must be faced if reproductive medicine is to reflect the emphasis on care for the person over pursuit of the disease, as we earlier advocated. Even more than with other courses of treatment where the fragility of the body points to the limits of effort, there is no objective point in infertility treatment at which it is clear that treatment will not work. There is always another cycle, another possibility along the spectrum of treatment options. The result, as we saw, is that patients sometimes cannot quit until they have simply exhausted all of their resources and their patience. The open-ended character of infertility is a component in the construction of infertility as a crisis. It is also part of the risk reproductive technologies pose to an already burdened health care budget. Because societal resources are finite and the good care of persons is at issue, the acceptance of limits must be as prominent a concern for distributive justice as the prior question of access.

Various possibilities have been proposed for setting limits. The medical model could be employed even more narrowly than it has been employed here, so that coverage is guaranteed only for the diagnosis and treatment of "correctable medical conditions." Under that principle, procedures such as the surgical repair of an obstructed fallopian tube would be included; IVF for male factor infertility would be excluded. We have already discussed the problems with such a standard. Applying it across the board would entail denying access to a variety of therapies and services aimed at compensating for impairments that cannot be corrected. Put another way, it would justify denying care in ways we have identified as important, the sort of caring we do when we help persons overcome obstacles to participation in the life of the community.

Limits could be imposed in the form of maximum benefits to be paid out for the treatment of any particular patient. Legislation enacted in Arkansas in 1987, for example, mandates coverage for infertility treatment up to a lifetime maximum of $15,000; Hawaii mandates a one-time-only benefit for all outpatient expenses arising from IVF.[24] Setting maximum limits for the treatment of particular health problems makes some sense as a way of directing the responsible use of resources. Any plan for guaranteeing universal access in the United States would have to pay attention to both overall and treatment specific expenditures. Setting limits on the treatment of infertility in the form of a maximum or one-time-only benefit, however, poses certain problems, as we have already seen. This type of cost control may encourage patients and physicians to move prematurely to sophisticated treatment or to use dangerously aggressive approaches to treatment in order to maximize chances of success. If discouraging irresponsibility, for example, the transfer of multiple viable embryos in IVF, is one of the goals of bringing reproductive medicine under scrutiny, we should be wary of the potential of this way of fixing limits to undercut that effort.

The approach most compatible with the framework of our discussion is one that makes limits treatment specific. For example, Illinois's mandate limits attempts at IVF for primary infertility to four complete oocyte retrievals. If initial treatment results in a live birth, two complete cycles are covered for a second attempt. The guarantee of four attempts at IVF may be too generous to advocate as a general rule. But limiting the number of cycles of IVF that will be reimbursed has the virtue of allowing for clinical discretion while giving weight to the reality of diminished returns. More than one cycle of IVF might be needed to achieve a pregnancy safely, but the chances of a successful outcome decline dramatically after four attempts. In addition to the relation between the number of attempts and the chances of success, other considerations might be brought to bear in setting limits. Success rates by age for particular treatments, for example, might be taken into account in determining a continuum of treatment levels. Four attempts may be reasonable for younger patients but irresponsible for older patients. Requiring patients to try less expensive treatment unless it is obvious that it will fail might also be a component of a treatment-specific framework. Questions like how many cycles of fertility drugs to require or whether an attempt or two at artificial insemination is appropriate before turning to IVF are complex and the answers are likely to keep changing as more is learned about the effectiveness of various procedures. The important point is that a treatment-specific methodology for setting limits allows a community to ask not only "How much are we spending?" but "What are we accomplishing?" It also recognizes the value of assisted reproduction for individuals without ignoring the absence of clear internal limits on the pursuit of fertility, a problem that extends beyond cost containment.

I have not attempted to articulate a policy for allocating infertility treatment within health care systems. Doing so would require far more attention to specific detail than would be desirable here. Rather, I have suggested a way of framing the determination of limits that aims at fostering the good care of infertile patients while discouraging the irresponsible or dangerous use of assisted reproductive technologies. One-time-only or maximum benefit approaches are less messy than the treatment-specific approach. What is gained in the latter, however, is important: the ability to take into account the particular needs of individual patients along a reasonable and prudent continuum of care.

Conclusion

We have tried in this chapter to sketch a broad framework for determining what equitable access might mean under conditions of limited resources. Throughout, the importance of caring well for individuals has been held in tension with the necessity of tempering the goals of reproductive medicine with realism and responsibility. Underlying the argument for a rationed approach to the treatment of infertility is a commitment to the common good that carries with it certain assumptions about the need for social transformation. In an ethic of the common good, seeking a way to bring accountability for the poor and the powerless into the debate over access to infertility treatment is just one part of calling the overall health care system to responsibility. The kind of reorientation of priorities for reproductive medicine being suggested here, from servicing consumer demands to meeting common needs, is one that must eventually take place on a societal and institutional level. It will be necessary, across the board, to probe the borders between overcoming obstacles and denying finitude, between identifying disabilities that inhibit participation and stigmatizing persons, and between curing and caring—all the complex and utterly central distinctions with which we have been concerned. It will be necessary to let go of some aspirations heretofore unquestioned—the hope to push back the boundaries of age, for example, or to treat each patient to the limits of one's skill—if we are to make possible a more equitable distribution of resources, to bring those now marginalized in the system to the center.

But obligations of accountability to the common good are personal as well as social and systemic. The questions that must be raised with respect to goals and priorities in reproductive medicine, in the health care system, and in the design of social institutions are also those that individuals must ask of their own choices. Recall Pieper's observation that the demands of distributive justice do not pertain only to those entrusted with the authority to distribute the goods of the community. The ruled also realize distributive justice as they "are contented by a just distribution." There are many different things that being "contented by a just distribution" might mean in the context of choices about fertility. It might mean simply that one accepts that there are limits to the community's obligation to assist in the pursuit of biological parenting and learns to live within them. Or it might mean the ability to recognize internal constraints on what ought to be asked of medicine in the attempt to overcome infertility. It might mean, in other words, the willingness to forgo therapies that threaten to place a great burden on the community with questionable benefit or that can be provided only at the cost of meeting the fundamental needs of others. Yet another possibility is that we are "contented" when we can choose to say no to assisted reproductive technology all together, redirecting the quest for a pregnancy into the creation of a welcoming heart for an already existing child in need of parents.

Discussions of health care reform seldom talk about how to cultivate contentment. Yet, if all that we have said about the need to question the demands we place on medicine today is correct, the ability to walk away, to live with sufficient rather than optimal care when justice for all requires it, is a necessary skill. The virtue of contentment may be especially important for those struggling with infertility. For all the reasons we have discussed, not all that can be done to overcome infertility should be done; not all that is available is either good or responsible medicine. But it is also, again for all the reasons we have named, excruciatingly difficult to say "no more" when more exists.

To overcome the loss of biological reproduction through opening one's home to a child no one else wants or by redirecting the drive for generativity into service to others is in the end to be able to "enlarge oneself" so that personal suffering embraces the community rather than shuts it out. It is as important to create conditions under which that capacity can be cultivated, and under which a healthy and responsible decision can be made not to pursue artificial reproduction, as it is to allow a place for infertility treatment in the assessment of health care priorities.

The freedom with which individuals, especially women, are able to recognize internal limits to appropriate care or to choose alternatives to advanced fertility treatment depends, however, upon the willingness of the community to understand and address their loss. In the final chapter, we will examine the failure of faith communities to recognize the crisis posed by infertility. The price, we will see, is the unrealized promise of a healing, self-enlarging spirituality.

NOTES

1 *Pacem in Terris* contains the most comprehensive (and in most estima-
tions, the most representative) delineation of human rights in the modern
Catholic social tradition. Here John XXIII argues that every human person, by virtue of her capacities for intelligence and free will, has a right
to life, bodily integrity, food, shelter, rest, medical care, and necessary social services, and the right to security in periods of illness, unemployment, and widowhood. A just society, he goes on, also protects a range of
social or cultural rights, for example the right to freedom of communication, to pursuit of art and of education, freedom of conscience and religious worship, and the right to found and support a family, as well as a
range of economic and political rights, including the right to private property and a living wage, and the rights of assembly and freedom of movement. Pope John XXIII, *Pacem in Terris* (April 11, 1963) 11–14, in *The
Gospel of Peace and Justice: Catholic Social Teaching since Pope John,*
presented by Joseph Gremillion (Maryknoll, N.Y.: Orbis Books, 1976),
203–09.
2 Charles Dougherty, *Back to Reform* (New York: Oxford University Press,
1996).
3 Martha C. Nussbaum, *Sex and Social Justice* (New York: Oxford University Press, 1999), 43.
4 Catholic Health Association, *With Justice for All? The Ethics of Health
Care Rationing* (St. Louis: The Catholic Health Association of the United
States, 1991), 16.
5 Ibid., 15.
6 Gene Outka, "Social Justice and Equal Access to Health Care," in *On
Moral Medicine: Theological Perspectives in Medical Ethics*, edited by
Stephen Lammers and Allan Verhey (Grand Rapids, Mich.: Eerdmans Publishing Co., 1988), 952.

7 President's Commission for the Study of Ethical Problems in Medicine and Biomedical and Behavioral Research, *Securing Access to Health Care* (Washington, D.C.: Government Printing Office, 1983).

8 Philip S. Keane, S.S., *Health Care Reform: A Catholic View* (Mahwah, N.J.: Paulist Press, 1993), 184.

9 Allen Buchanan, "An Ethical Evaluation of Health Care in the United States," *Contemporary Issues in Bioethics*, 4th edition, edited by Tom L. Beauchamp and LeRoy Walters (Belmont, Calif: Wadsworth Publishing Co., 1994), 727.

10 Allen Buchanan, "The Right to a Decent Minimum of Health Care," in *Contemporary Issues in Bioethics,* 4th edition, edited by Tom L. Beauchamp and LeRoy Walters (Belmont, Calif.: Wadsworth Publishing Co., 1994), 697.

11 Philip Keane, *Health Care Reform*, 142.

12 "The Goals of Medicine: Setting New Priorities," *Hastings Center Report* 26, no. 6, special supplement (1996), S9.

13 Martha Nussbaum, *Sex and Social Justice*, 39.

14 Daniel Callahan, *What Kind of Life? The Limits of Medical Progress* (New York: Simon and Schuster, 1990), 175–85.

15 Ibid., 190–91.

16 Ibid.

17 Ibid., 180–81.

18 Beverly Wildung Harrison, "Theological Reflection in the Struggle for Liberation," in *Making the Connection: Essays in Feminist Social Theory,* edited by Carol S. Robb (Boston: Beacon Press, 1985), 255.

19 M. Griffin and W. F. Panak, "The Economic Cost of Infertility-Related Services: An Examination of the Massachusetts Infertility Insurance Mandate," *Fertility and Sterility* 70, no. 1 (1998): 22–29.

20 See Norman Daniels, *Just Heath Care* (Cambridge: Cambridge University Press, 1985), 104–05.

21 Many centers report never having had a successful IVF pregnancy after age 45 without the use of donor eggs.

22 See M. Van Thiel, E. Mantadakis, and M. Vekemans, "A Psychological Study, Using Interviews and Projective Tests, of Patients Seeking Anonymous Donor Artificial Insemination," *Journal de Gynecologie, Obstetrique et Biologie de la Reproduction* (Paris) 1990, 19, no. 7: 823–28; D. M. Berger, A. Eisen, J. Shuber, and K. F. Doody, "Psychological Patterns in Donor Insemination Couples," *Canadian Journal of Psychiatry* (December 31, 1986), 818–23; J. Kremer, B. W. Frijling, and J. L. Nass, "Psychological Aspects of Parenthood by AID," *Lancet* 7, no. 1 (March 1984): 628. In general, controlled studies of the AID experience show a high rate of satisfaction with AID and no greater rate of marital discord or parenting problems in AID recipient couples than in populations conceiving normally.

See K. R. Daniels, W. R. Gillett, and G. P. Herbison, "Successful Donor Insemination and Its Impact on Recipients," *Journal of Psychosomatic Obstetrics and Gynaecology,* 17 no. 3 (September 1996): 129–34; A. McWhinnie, "A Study of Parenting of IVF and DI Children," *Medicine and Law* 14, no. 7–8 (1995): 501–08; L. R. Schover, R. L. Collins, and S. Richards, "Psychological Aspects of Donor Insemination: Evaluation and Follow-up of Recipient Couples," *Fertility and Sterility* 57, no. 3 (March 1992): 583–90.

23 It may be, of course, that women who participate in online discussion groups devoted to lending support for the decision to undergo donor-assisted reproduction are more likely to find the experience positive than women who do not. In any case, the articulated experience of such women should not be discounted, even if we should be modest in the conclusions we draw from it.

24 Information provided by the Office of Government Relations of the American Fertility Society (now the American Society for Reproductive Medicine), April 1992.

CHAPTER SIX

FAITH AND INFERTILITY

"I don't long for a baby anymore. I long to be free of the longing."

—Anonymous, in private communication

Last December a regular member of a web-based infertility support group wrote that although she really wanted to attend church services during Advent, she planned to stay away. Her husband had finally convinced her not to go. Rather than finding comfort there, he argued, she seemed only to come home sadder. With so many references to childbirth and family during the Christmas season, he worried that her going to church would set them further back in their efforts to move beyond infertility.

It is not unusual to hear infertility patients express deep ambivalence about religion. As Arthur Greil observed, there is often a bargaining stage in infertility, something like the behavior observed in patients who have received a terminal diagnosis, in which promises are made to God in exchange for a different outcome.[1] The infertile light candles, say special prayers, wear medals and amulets, in the hope of winning God's favor in the conception lottery. Yet, often underlying the novenas to St. Jude and the prayers of atonement for past sins is a simmering anger at a God who "opens and closes wombs at will" and at a church that prizes the ability to bear children while seeming to offer little sustenance to those who by nature or circumstance are denied the chance.

If those who are struggling with infertility turn to the church only to come home sadder or angrier, the faith community has missed an important opportunity. As we have seen, infertility can pose a serious life crisis, particularly for women. Facing the fact that one will never conceive or bear children is not just an experience of profound disappointment. Rather, it feels like a kind of "dying," a loss of both an envisioned future and a possible self, a potential role and a longed-for relationship. It is a death that occurs without a body or a funeral, a death without a ritual or a ceremony to mark it.[2] Infertility is rarely recognized as such a crisis, however, and even when it is, it is treated largely as a medical or social crisis. It is seldom recognized as a spiritual crisis, a deep confrontation of meaning and belief. Yet, it is precisely when infertility is acknowledged as questioning one's very understanding of oneself and one's place in the universe that the pain and disappointment of infertility can become an opportunity for personal and spiritual growth. Indeed, it is only when infertility is seen as a spiritual crisis that it can initiate a *spiritual quest*, an occasion for "a blossoming of self far more rewarding than mere endurance."[3]

In the same way, it is when the threat to the integrity of the self posed by a diagnosis of infertility is addressed that it becomes possible to say no to medical interventions that have become pointless or destructive to persons or relationships. As Eric Cassell showed in the case of terminal illness, the ability to accept the limits of mortality in a healthy way depends upon having transcended the suffering caused by what the ill or dying person "loses in relation to the world of objects, events and relationships."[4] When we fail to understand and treat infertility as a spiritual crisis, we overlook the resources that exist within our religious tradition for enabling self-transformation within those losses and for helping individuals move to a posture in which ceasing medical treatment does not mean abandoning hope. We lose the chance to make visible alternative possibilities for family relationship in the tradition's rich understanding of membership in the body of Christ. We miss the particular occasion for discipleship presented in the unfulfilled desire for a child. Just as it is possible to die healed, so it is possible to let go of the pursuit of fertility and to embrace adoption or childlessness. But to do either, one needs to come to peace with a redefinition of the self against a horizon now recast by illness or infertility. Given the potential of infertility treatment to become an emotional and financial trap, it is especially tragic if the infertile cannot find a place within the spiritual and liturgical life of the church in which to seek that peace.

The question for this final chapter, then, is how to construct a spirituality for growth or transcendence through infertility. What theological and liturgical resources exist for creating conditions in which it is possible both to learn and to share the lessons infertility teaches about finitude and humility? What would it mean, for example, to see the liturgical and pastoral life of the church as a context for acquiring the grace to live into involuntary childlessness with hope and dignity?

Mixed Messages and Missed Opportunities

There are many references to infertility in Scripture.[5] The birth of a son to a long-infertile or "barren" wife is a familiar symbol of God's favor. Isaac is born to Abraham, signifying both Abraham's reward for his fidelity and Yahweh's guarantee of a viable future for Israel. Through the child, the covenant is established; Sarah (at ninety) becomes not only an improbable mother, but the "mother of nations" (Gen. 17:15–21). In turn, the Lord grants Isaac's prayer and the barren Rebekah gives birth to Esau and Jacob (Gen. 25:21). Vowing to dedicate her child to God if only God would grant her a son, Hannah is finally "remembered," and she bears Samuel (1 Sam. 9–11; 19–20). Like Abraham and Sarah, the righteous Zechariah and Elizabeth of the New Testament, well beyond childbearing years, are sent a son who is to be "great before the Lord," whose birth in joy and wonder is a foretaste of the redemptive events to come (Luke 1:8–19). The long-awaited child, born to this woman now at the "end" of her life, is testimony indeed that "with God, nothing will be impossible" (Luke 1:36–37).

Barrenness plays different roles in the biblical texts. Sometimes it stands as a sign of God's judgment. Only rarely does God "close wombs" in an act of explicit punishment, as in Genesis 20:1–18.[6] But fertility is a blessing, as the psalmist reminds his listeners: "Lo, sons are a heritage from the Lord, the fruit of the womb a reward" (Ps. 127:3). By inference, barrenness is a curse: As the Lord gives abundantly to those He favors, so it seems He withholds or withdraws from those He rebukes (Deut. 7:12–15). In other places, barrenness functions as a pretext for a miraculous intervention. The lifelong infertility of Sarah and Elizabeth seems merely to lay the scene for the appearance of the extraordinary child; the improbability of such a birth underscoring the power of God, which knows not even natural limits. Still at other times, barrenness appears as sheer mystery. We are never told why God "remembered" Rachel (Gen. 30:22) or Hannah (1 Sam. 1:19) or, indeed, why they were forgotten in the first place.

As Phyllis Trible argues in *God and the Rhetoric of Sexuality*, in some sense barrenness is an extrinsic phenomenon in the biblical texts. The womb is "a physical object on which the deity acts. Control of it belongs neither to women nor to their husbands, neither to the fetus nor to society. Only God closes and opens wombs in judgment, in blessing, and in mystery."[7] At the same time, the individual or personal suffering associated with barrenness is clearly visible. Infertility is linked to illness and famine in the promises of Sinai: "You shall serve the Lord your God, and I will bless your bread and water; and I will take sickness away from the midst of you. None shall cast her young or be barren in your land. I will fulfill the number of your days" (Exod. 23:25–26). The barren woman is an object of derision, for the inability to conceive and bear children—and in particular, to bear sons—is assumed to lie with her. We get glimpses of the pain of infertility in Rachel's cry to Jacob: "Give me children, or I shall die!" (Gen. 30:2); in Issac's plea to Yahweh on behalf of his wife (Gen. 25:21); and in the psalmist's identification of the barren woman with the poorest of the poor: "He raises the poor from the dust, and lifts the needy from the ash heap, to make them sit with princes. . . . He gives the barren woman a home, making her the joyous mother of children" (Ps. 113). The most poignant glimpse is the picture of Hannah in the first book of Samuel. The second wife of Elkanah, she is taunted, year after year, by her rival because "the Lord had closed her womb" (1 Sam 1:6). Rising in the temple, she prays to Yahweh "in the bitterness of her soul": "O Lord of Hosts, if thou wilt indeed look on the affliction of thy maidservant, and remember me, and not forget thy maidservant, but wilt give to thy maidservant a son, then I will give him to the Lord all the days of his life, and no razor shall touch his head" (1 Sam. 12). So great is her distress that she is mistaken by the priest Eli for drunk. "No, my lord," Hannah explains, "I am a woman sorely troubled; I have drunk neither wine nor strong drink, but I have been pouring out my soul before the Lord. Do not regard your maidservant as a base woman, for all along I have been speaking out of my great anxiety and vexation" (1 Sam. 1:9–17).

It would seem that Western religious traditions shaped by sacred texts so rich in the imagery of fertility and infertility would provide a natural context in which to come to terms with the suffering occasioned by infertility. But Greil's study of American infertile couples showed instead that it is extremely difficult for infertile believers to draw on their religious faith in trying to make sense of infertility. He found that "both husbands and wives who used [religious] language spontaneously seemed *more* likely to find infertility a threat to meaning than those who did not; likewise, both wives and husbands who reported attending religious services regularly were more likely to see infertility as a threat to meaning than those who did not." Some couples reported drawing strength from the social relationships they enjoyed within their faith communities, but they were far outnumbered by those who viewed religious affiliation as one more obstacle to be overcome in their attempt to deal with their infertility. Overall, he concluded, "religion [did] not provide most couples in my sample with resources upon which they can call to explain to themselves their experience of suffering."[8]

Why is it that many people, many Christians, who are dealing with infertility have difficulty finding solace and usable wisdom in religion? One reason is that for all its relative visibility in the Bible, infertility is an invisible reality in most religious congregations. Last December, the priest in my family's parish prayed for all families during the liturgy for the feast of the Holy Family, including families undergoing divorce and blended and nontraditional families. Afterward, a friend told me how grateful she felt, as the mother of a blended family (a family with step-children), to have been mentioned. Never could she remember a celebrant even recognizing the existence of blended families. As she described her feelings of marginalization, especially on occasions where special attention is given to family life, I thought of the many times in which, on similar occasions, I waited in vain to hear any mention of those in the congregation who were experiencing difficulty in beginning or building a family. I thought, in particular, of the many Mother's Day liturgies I have attended. It is difficult to describe just how painful it can be for an infertile woman to be surrounded by the celebration of motherhood. Yet, I cannot recall a single time in which the pain of longing for parenthood was acknowledged liturgically alongside the joy and struggles of its realization.

My experience is limited to Roman Catholic congregations, where pastoral insensitivity to issues of infertility is no doubt exacerbated by an all-male, celibate clergy. However, there is ample anecdotal testimony from infertile women to suggest that the experience of invisibility is not limited to Catholic congregations nor to male clergy. Indeed, there is a heavily visited website named "Hannah's Prayer" that provides online spiritual resources for Christians dealing with issues of infertility and pregnancy loss as well as liturgical resources for congregations.[9] The site was created, according to its founders, to fill a lacuna in support systems for those looking for help in drawing on their Christian faith in coping with infertility. Its several sections devoted to "advice for pastors, clergy and church leaders" attest to their readers' experience of finding little in their communities of faith to encourage them in dealing creatively with their feelings of frustration or in learning how to pray "from the depths of their grief and resentment."

Another reason why religion can be more of an obstacle than a pathway to healing for the infertile is the ambiguous and somewhat contradictory character of fertility in religious literature. In the Roman Catholic tradition, for example, procreation is treated as one of the primary goods of marriage. As the Catechism of the Catholic Church teaches: "Fecundity is a gift, an end of marriage, for conjugal love naturally tends to be fruitful. A child does not come from outside as something added on to the mutual love of the spouses, but springs from the very heart of the mutual giving, as its fruit and fulfillment."[10] The tradition recognizes what many infertile couples already believe passionately: that reproduction "completes" or "embodies" an intimate relationship. To bring forth a child who is "flesh of our flesh" symbolizes the joining of their separate lives in a concrete and living way. The act of reproducing moves the relationship to a new level, not only symbolically but also practically, as the couple makes the transition to an all-encompassing, necessarily responsible or outwardly focused intimacy. That marital love should be "completed" in this way is treated not just as a value in the tradition but as a kind of natural fact. Although the supposition that each and every sexual act must be open to reproduction has come increasingly under attack, it is nonetheless assumed in Catholic sexual ethics that reproduction is a primary, "essential" end of sexual expression. Even if the good of biological reproduction ought to give way to other goods or values in a particular case, that sexual intimacy inclines toward generativity is taken (in a positive sense) as a given.

In much the same way, the language of lay vocation in the Catholic tradition assumes the centrality of reproduction in marriage. In the apostolic letter *Mulieris Dignitatem,* for example, Pope John Paul II links the capacity for reproduction with women's fundamental, universal vocation: "God entrusts the human being to [woman] in a special way . . . precisely by reason of their femininity—and this in a particular way determines their vocation."[11] Marriage is not, of course, necessary for salvation in the Catholic tradition. The vowed life has long been a valued (in some eras, a highly revered) alternative to marriage for both men and women.[12] When attention is turned to the specific role of the laity as Christians in the world, however, the descriptive categories employed center on the duties of marriage and family life. The family is extolled as a special site for the cultivation of moral and religious values. Parental responsibilities have both a personal and social function: "Married couples should regard it as their proper mission to transmit human life and to educate their children; they should realize that they are thereby cooperating with the love of God the creator and are, in a certain sense, its interpreters."[13] Feminist theologians have been sharply critical of the language of complementarity underlying discussions of the lay vocation, particularly in magisterial teaching.[14] To assume that women have a "natural vocation" to the home (and men to the social sphere) is problematic on many fronts, not the least of which is its use in justifying the exclusion of women from leadership roles in the church. Even its sharpest critics, however, do not reject the religious and social significance of "motherhood" or "fatherhood" nor their importance in the vocational identity of individuals. Indeed, it might be said that it is precisely because they recognize the magnitude of the task involved in bringing children into the world that feminist theologians insist that the role should be undertaken freely and in the light of genuine alternatives.

Alongside the priority of place given to reproduction and the parental role in the Roman Catholic tradition, however, is the tendency, as noted earlier, to speak of fertility in the language of "gift" and "blessing."[15] Insisting that children are the "gift" of a marriage rightly avoids the problematic categories of "right" and "entitlement" that dominate contemporary debates over the limits of procreative liberty. "Gift" or "blessing" imagery preserves the sense in which, in a theological context, the miracle of a new life is always a great and finally undeserved good and the sense in which children come into our care but are never things possessed. At the same time, when placed against the assumption that procreation is a natural and expected end or goal of fully realized sexual intimacy, "gift" or "blessing" language leaves infertile believers in a paradoxical and ultimately untenable position. On the one hand, they are encouraged to see their marital relationship as appropriately growing toward fullness or completion in the enterprise of parenthood and to see themselves as adult Christians, at least in part, in light of the contributions they will make as Christian parents. On the other hand, they have no right to expect that they will be able to partake in this "expected" role. Children are a gift, seemingly distributed without regard for readiness, deservingness, or fitness. The frustration many infertile Catholics express concerning *Donum Vitae's* analysis of reproductive technology springs from the feeling that they are receiving a double-message: fertility is a great value to be expressed and cultivated *except* in the case of the infertile; for them, it is merely another good that God has, for whatever reasons, chosen not to grant their marriage, a missing blessing which can be readily compensated for with a "generous spirit."

Yet another reason why, for many people, religion provides little comfort in the journey through infertility is suggested in the brief survey of biblical references to barrenness above. The interwoven symbolisms of judgment, blessing, and mystery yield a confusing answer to the suffering occasioned by infertility. As we have seen, infertile women, in particular, tend, at least at a certain stage in the process, to blame themselves for their inability to conceive or bear a child. They try to gain power in the face of powerlessness by becoming the agent of their own suffering. Earlier failures of judgment or volition, a previous short-sightedness, or youthful self-centeredness account for their present anguish. The temptation to see infertility as a punishment is especially great for those women who have had a previous abortion or who have or had ambivalent feelings about the use of birth control. Alice Domar, director of the Mind/Body Center for Women's Health at Boston's Beth Israel Deaconess Hospital, observes that, in her experience, "the very religious patients or the ones brought up in the most religious homes have the hardest time with infertility. Women who truly believe that they are being punished for their sins, who believe in a punitive God, will be the worst off."[16]

However, efforts to levy blame (even self-blame) for conditions such as infertility are as ultimately unsatisfying as they are natural. For one thing, it is often difficult to identify the exact etiology of infertility. Moreover, the role of any particular set of choices (for example, to postpone childbearing) is frequently ambiguous and impossible to trace in the manner of cause and effect or in a way that makes it easy to fix blame. However attractive it might be to find an answer to the questions of meaning posed by infertility in an account of God's judgment, it is extremely difficult in the end to take seriously the conclusion that infertility is a punishment for some past misdeeds or misplaced desires.[17] The nightly news is full of accounts of unwanted and badly cared for children, born to seemingly "undeserving" mothers and fathers. How is it that these infertile women and men, who understand better than anyone how precious is the life of a child, are pointedly passed over when the blessing of children is elsewhere so freely and apparently indiscriminately bestowed? What exactly did they do that warrants such a devastating punishment?

To see infertility as a mystery is perhaps a better place to begin in articulating a theological response to the infertility crisis. Accepting the belief that "bad things sometimes happen to good people" does not require being able to explain infertility, either in terms of individual agency or divine judgment. At the same time, infertility can be "handed over" into the broad embrace of God's providence, where all that is and all that occurs, if not eventually explained, still falls under the wisdom and love of a gracious creator.

Infertility as mystery is not, however, that much more satisfying as theodicy than infertility as punishment. For one thing, while Scripture is rich with models of hope and reward (Hannah's anguished and angry cry does not finally go unheeded), we are hard-pressed to find models for living with unresolved infertility. It is easier, as Greil observed, for couples who have adopted or finally had a child to find answers to their suffering in the promise-patience-blessing stories of the miraculous children of Scripture than for those who are in the midst of the journey through infertility.[18] Yet, that is where the deepest challenge of meaning lies, precisely in the process of coming to terms with infertility, where what is most important is the ability to make self- and life-affirming decisions about how to address infertility and how far to go in pursuing parenthood medically. To conclude that there is no theological answer for infertility save that it is a mystery may not only be ultimately disappointing as an answer but may play directly into the hands of contemporary "medical" or "scientific" theodicies. From the standpoint of reproductive medicine, impaired reproduction is not a mystery to be pondered but a technical problem in need of a technical solution. In such circumstances, argues Greil,

traditional theodicies which counsel stoicism in the face of the inevitable [or unexplainable] may lose ground to the impatient theodicy implied by the medical model. According to the medical model, suffering is not something to be understood but rather something to be conquered. Explanations that rely on such concepts as "God's will" cannot be convincing when we believe as strongly as we do in the human ability to pull ourselves out of our condition through technical knowledge.[19]

If at least some of what we hope for in religious faith is the strength, when necessary, to cease treatment without abandoning hope or to accept other outlets for generativity, the answer that the suffering occasioned by infertility is simply a mystery does little more to promote a healthy resolution of the crisis than the answer that the suffering occasioned by infertility is a punishment for something one has done. This is especially so in the absence of models for living what is often a difficult and life-defining mystery such as this faithfully.

The difficulties infertile believers encounter in drawing a usable or healing wisdom from faith traditions stem both from how we treat infertility within communities of faith and how we talk about infertility in theological terms. Constructing a healing or transcendent spirituality, therefore, includes practical or pastoral strategies as well as theological reconstruction.

Creating a Context

If infertile believers find religious services "among the most painful times in their week"[20] in large part because they feel invisible or marginalized within faith communities that place a great deal of emphasis on families and family life, much could be done to create opportunities for healing simply by "attending to the moment." With sensitivity on the part of the celebrant, the same liturgical events that we now use for celebrating and supporting families could become opportunities for making the invisible struggle of the infertile visible. By including a prayer for all those who want to be mothers or fathers and are experiencing difficulty, for example, the liturgical celebrations of Mother's Day and Father's Day could be both a "teachable moment" for the congregation and an opportunity for the expression of solidarity.[21] Simply by acknowledging the varied experiences of family present in any faith community, our observances of the feast of the Holy Family could become occasions for inviting in those who feel on the margins rather than merely retracing the lines of inclusion and exclusion. Attention to the language and symbols we use in the public rituals and sermons marking religiously important moments of family life, such as baptisms, first communions, and confirmations, and an effort to listen from the perspective of those who are currently struggling with some aspect of family could go far in easing the pain of those who experience those events as excruciating.

In *Dealing with Infertility: A Guide for Catholics*, Julie Kelemen gives a good illustration of how becoming aware of those on the margins can transform an isolating moment to a healing moment:

> *For several consecutive weeks, our parish bulletin carried an announcement about a special blessing of expectant parents planned for all masses on an upcoming Sunday. I looked forward to this blessing since I knew that we would probably be adoptive parents some day. But when the actual Mass and blessing came, and I saw the other couples walk to the front of the church for their special blessing, I froze. I feared that the deacon would place his hands over the women's bellies to "bless the fruits of their wombs." If that were to happen, I knew I would have to walk away because there would never be a child inside me. I could not walk forward and felt hurt that my church may not have meant this blessing for my husband and me at all.[22]*

After Mass, Kelemen and her husband approached the deacon and explained why they did not come forward. They asked if they, too, could be given the medals of St. Gerard Majella and St. Joseph (patron saints of expectant mothers and fathers) he had given to the other couples. The deacon explained that he had not meant to exclude adopting parents, but neither had it occurred to him to mention them. Kelemen reported that after that incident, announcements concerning events for expectant parents also included "adopting parents." Although Kelemen does not suggest it, it might have been important to at least some people in that congregation to have also included "hopeful parents" in the invitation to blessing.

It is also possible to create moments for reaching out to the infertile within the liturgical year. The Cedar Park Assemblies of God Church in Bothell, Washington, sets aside Presentation Sunday each year for a special blessing for infertile couples. In 1998, twenty parishes in Bothell joined Cedar Park in inviting those who were suffering infertility or pregnancy loss to come together to pray and to experience the support of the community.[23] Widely publicized, Presentation Sunday calls attention to the reality of infertility within congregations and gives public witness to the possibilities for encountering infertility as a spiritual journey. Although many people come to such a service to pray for a miracle, it also provides a context for exploring the challenge of living faithfully in the absence of miracles.

Crisis events like miscarriages open up opportunities for addressing infertility and pregnancy loss as moments of spiritual anguish and potential growth. The importance of developing ways to ritualize pregnancy loss cannot be underestimated, especially in religious traditions that stress that life begins at conception. Where there is no burial, no memorializing of a named life, no final commendation, it can be extremely difficult for couples who believe they have lost a child, not just a pregnancy, to come to terms with the event. Hannah's Prayer offers helpful examples of services that can be used in cases of early pregnancy loss, which invite parents to express their grief and to put closure on the pregnancy publicly and, with the support of the community, to entrust their child to God's care.[24] Models can also be found in feminist rituals for marking passages in women's lives. Recovering spiritually from miscarriage involves both grieving the loss of a potential child and reclaiming one's body or refocusing one's life force. Burying the possible names of a lost fetus or planting a tree signifying the ended pregnancy can be powerful ways of symbolically expressing the death of the pregnancy and the otherwise silent transition from pregnant to no longer pregnant.

It would also be valuable to develop religious rituals for marking the end of aggressive infertility treatment. To give up on the dream of a biologically related child or the dream of parenting itself is, as we have seen, a kind of death, which, like other deaths, cries out for a public acknowledgment of mourning. For many people, it is difficult to give up on scientific power without coming to embrace another sort of power—the power of God or a new power within oneself. A ritual for moving on might symbolize the transition through prayer from a primary reliance on the promise of medicine to a new level of reliance on the promises of God. Through a symbolic burying of one's hopes for parenthood (for example, burying the names one hoped to give one's children or the fantasies one had about the looks or personalities of future children), such a ritual could also enact or make visible the necessary transition from living cycle-to-cycle to living into the rest of reconceived life.

Attending to the moments which make visible or invisible the experience of infertility and pregnancy loss within a faith community and creating moments for gathering liturgical resources in the service of healing are both important ways of addressing the spiritual dimensions of what we have called the infertility crisis. But the more challenging question posed by the experience of infertile couples in the church is what role faith might play in the journey to *come to terms* with infertility. What, if anything, can we say theologically to the woman who "longs to be free of the longing"?

From Spiritual Crisis to Spiritual Quest

As we have seen, there are ample references to barrenness in Scripture. But, as we have also seen, the infertile woman seeking comfort in Scripture comes away with a confusing picture. Is she to regard her infertility as mystery or punishment? May she, must she, continue to count on a miracle? Is it patience or persistence that finally gets God's attention?

In what follows, we will trace a spiritual path that begins in a very different place than where we usually begin when we think about faith and infertility. It begins not with the stories of miraculous births, but in the early chapters of Luke:

> *As he went, the people pressed round him. And a woman who had a flow of blood for twelve years and could not be healed by anyone, came up behind him, and touched the fringe of his garment; and immediately, her flow of blood ceased. And Jesus said, "Who was it that touched me?" When all denied it, Peter said, "Master, the multitudes surround you and press upon you!" But Jesus said, "Some one touched me; for I perceive that power has gone forth from me." And when the woman saw that she was not hidden, she came trembling, and falling down before him declared in the presence of all the people why she had touched him and how she had been immediately healed. And he said to her, "Daughter, your faith has made you well; go in peace." (Luke 8:42–48)*

The story of the hemorrhaging woman lacks the satisfying completeness of Hannah's story. It has none of the drama of her anguished cry in the temple or the joyous resolution in the birth of Samuel. And it is precisely its incompleteness that makes it a powerful text for reflecting on the possibilities for spiritual healing within the experience of infertility. There are plenty of miracle tales in today's reproductive medicine, at least for those willing and able to try anything and spend anything, But the day-to-day, month-to-month reality of infertility is more often a narrative of frustration and failure, of disappointment after disappointment, played out in a dramatic way in the infertile woman's body. She is, like the hemorrhaging woman, the unwilling subject of a "flow" that cannot be stopped. Her menstrual period comes on schedule, often the first dreaded sign that efforts to conceive have failed. Infertility is an affront to power over self at the most intimate level. Not only is her body not in her control, but the unsuccessful struggle to conceive becomes in her a battle in which, as one woman put it starkly,

> *she is defeated by herself, by her own body, puking its blood and pain at the end of each month, the temperature chart declining steeply and her plans and projects and designs decreasing with the lowered heat of her body.*[25]

And like the hemorrhaging woman, her wound is not visible. She, too, is isolated, her pain hidden within the multitudes of a fertile world.

What can we learn from Luke's hemorrhaging woman? Jan Rehner argues that healing from infertility begins with a reconception of the self:

> *For those women who have wandered in the labyrinth of infertility or whose lives will never fit the narratives of mother and child, there is a necessity for a* "new seeing or revelation of what is, which then requires a new naming of self and world." *There needs to be, in short, a new story, the creation of an alternate vision of self that is not a negation, but a statement of the wholeness and fulfillment of other equally viable possibilities.*[26]

This "new naming" of the self is not a denial of infertility, nor is it merely a matter of throwing oneself into other projects, as infertile couples are often encouraged to do. Rather, the possibility of constructing an "alternate vision of the self that is not a negation" follows from facing directly the feelings of grief, inferiority, anger, and so on, that are a central part of the experience of infertility. It is precisely in "coming out of the crowd" with the woman in Luke's gospel, in accepting infertility as a dimension of one's being that has been internalized as defect, handicap, self-abnegation that the process of integrating infertility as a dimension of one's whole person, one's womanhood can begin. "To say aloud and to believe, when it can no longer be resisted, 'I cannot bear children,' is to begin to be free."[27]

The "new seeing" or revelation that makes possible a "new naming" involves coming to terms with what infertility has taken from one's life, facing the way in which infertility represents the collapse of a "sustaining life purpose," or in Cassell's terms, the catastrophic loss of the self in relation to "objects, events and relationships."[28] It also involves seeing beyond what has been lost to what remains and coming to understand how what remains is enriched by what has been lost. Although feminist theologians have not taken seriously enough the experience of infertile women, we can find resources in feminism for this movement from revelation to an alternate vision. Feminists have recognized the centrality of reproduction in women's lives, and despite a critical awareness of its often destructive social construction, have celebrated reproduction as a singular achievement of women. Feminist theory has affirmed the root of the suffering that infertile women experience: The ability to pass on the gift of life is an intrinsic part of how women understand and orient their lives. At the same time, feminism has vigorously resisted defining reproduction as the primary function, the only authentic achievement of women. Rather, "being women is the authentic achievement among women, living full lives based on self-identity, responsibility, autonomy."[29] Feminism has encouraged women to throw off the oppressive message that a woman's purpose in life is to reproduce and has demanded accountability for social and political arrangements that equate women's status with her ability to bear children. In celebrating a rich understanding of "woman," and a vision of feminine energy as a power not just for birth but for connection, growth, and transformation, feminism provides a framework for the deeper understanding of fertility or "fruitfulness" that is necessary in the healing process for infertile women. Rehner writes, "It is . . . this sense of our own beauty and sensuality and passion and right to be that infertile women need to feel and express. In denying our bodies, we den[ied] ourselves wisdom, joy and community."[30]

Those who have resolved the infertility crisis (whether or not they ever became parents) have learned how to tap into the vital energy that all human beings possess and of which the ability to impregnate or give birth is only one small manifestation. They have come in touch with the deep life-giving forces outside themselves and have grown to see the many possibilities for generativity in the lives they are now living. From denying and hating a body that will not make babies, they come to embrace a body as rich as ever in capacities for love, recreation, passion, and courage, only grown wiser now through suffering. Like AIDS patients who have successfully navigated the crisis posed by their diagnosis, they have come to see the altered life as nonetheless rich in possibilities. As Paulette Bates Alden puts it, they have let the other "anticipated" or "correct" life, go:

> *Having children was something we didn't get. . . . Life doesn't always give you what you expect or want, though it may give you different, possibly better things.*

> *I'm in the midst of my own life, and if it isn't the life I might have expected exactly, it is the life I have. I tend to think it's the life I've wanted,*

in spite of myself. I happen to like it. It seems to me a rich and blessed life. Every day I'm grateful for it.[31]

In some sense, those who successfully transcend the loss posed by infertility are those for whom the experience of infertility has become a kind of "spiritual pregnancy," an occasion for giving birth to a new understanding and appreciation of the self.[32]

Self-acceptance is a critical moment in the spiritual journey through infertility. So, too, is coming to a new relationship with God and with God's purposes for one's life. "The faith that will make us well" is not principally a relentless expectation of a miracle. Rather, it is the willingness to be "called out of the crowd" in our infirmity and touched by the God who is the source of all life and all energy. Feelings of anger at God are normal and even necessary to the process of healing. But equally necessary is the movement from asking: "What is God doing to me/us?" to "Where is God leading me/us?" Just as it is important to come to see the self-transforming possibilities within the experience of infertility, healing in a spiritual sense involves opening oneself to the possibilities for spiritual reawakening in the experience of suffering or loss.

Edmund Pellegrino and David Thomasma argue that the virtue of hope is necessary for genuine healing to take place—hope in God's friendship, God's mercy, God's ultimate design for our lives. Such a hope is not

a simple, romantic disavowal of the reality of suffering and dying. It does not require replacing the benefits of medical care, however limited they may be in some cases, with pious presumption that a miracle will occur. Christian hope recognizes that God may, indeed, work a miracle, but it also recognizes that his goodness and solicitude are there regardless of whether a miracle occurs. . . . Christian hope is not an invitation to unrealism or false expectations. It confronts the realities of the patient's predicament, but it directs the mind and heart to something much larger, the reality of God's presence in history, his promises to humanity, and his unfailing love for every one of his creatures.[33]

As this description suggests, a transformative spirituality in the face of infertility will not be built on the expectation of miracles (as important as it may be to the infertile not to lose confidence entirely in the possibility of an unexpected blessing) but on awareness of the constant companionship of God in the experience of infirmity, disappointment, or despair. As with the dying, the community of faith is called to embody this transcendent hope, not by piously denying the realities of infertility, but by becoming a site where the "something much larger" can be witnessed and the capacity to trust that all things, even our present sufferings, are working to good can be learned. When hope is grasped as an awareness of God's redeeming work within our experiences of illness or loss or despair, when it is not mistaken simply for a commitment to a certain outcome, it becomes possible for infertility to be the catalyst for a new and deeper relationship with God and the community. It also becomes possible to bring realistic expectations to medicine. Stopping treatment is abandoning hope only when success or failure is measured as the achievement of a certain result. When the experience of infertility is lived as an invitation to experience the mystery of God's care for us, God's infinite "motherhood" and "fatherhood," God's desire for our flourishing, it is not necessary to pursue "success" at the expense of the self. Indeed, it does not even make sense.

Luke's hemorrhaging woman leaves her encounter with Jesus cured. But the story is less about her finally finding help for her physical problem than it is about her coming out of the crowd and coming into the presence of a healing, transformative love. What those struggling with infertility need, and what we as communities of faith owe to them, is an inviting witness to the "something more" that lies beyond the limits of their loss. It is only then that we can turn faith or religion from "one more painful obstacle to resolving infertility" to a genuine source and context for healing.

Conclusions and the Work Yet to Be Done

Reflecting on the importance of Christian hope in cultivating an ethic of healthy restraint in medicine, Richard McCormick observed that the capacity to prayerfully accept our finitude in the face of aging or illness rests on a theology of dependence that has yet to be developed.[34] We have the resources in the Christian tradition's belief in life everlasting to counter today's temptation to chase a cure at all costs. But as a people of faith, we have not learned how to talk about the loss of independence or function as a moment of grace, nor, despite our acknowledgment of the realities of aging, disability and death within our communities, have we cultivated the virtues of patience, humility, and endurance.

We could make an analogous observation about the capacity to accept infertility's limits. There are resources in the Christian tradition for seeing infertility as an opportunity for personal and spiritual rebirth. But we have not developed a spirituality of involuntary childlessness through which the infertile could come to experience the "something beyond" in their suffering or through which their infertility could become a teacher of the meaning of "birth" or "generativity" for the community. We could also extend McCormick's critique to observe that in general we have not called forth models for faithful living into aging, death, or infertility within our communities. The late Cardinal Joseph Bernardin of Chicago gave a great gift to the Church in his honest, articulate, and courageous acceptance of his death from pancreatic cancer. In some parishes, women are forming "crone" groups to provide a context for the celebration of joyful and creative aging. But for the most part we create few opportunities for the aging, the dying, the disabled—in this case, the infertile—to show us how to do it with grace and fidelity.

The lack of a living "spirituality of limits" in our communities is an obstacle to retrieving the power of faith for healing in the context of infertility. There are other obstacles that ought to be acknowledged as well. As I noted earlier, the infertile receive a kind of double message about reproduction: having children is a great blessing, the *telos* of married life, and the most celebrated channel through which lay Catholics participate in the ministry of the church. But those who cannot have children are expected to be able quite easily to direct their desire for children to "other important [human] services," such as "adoption, various forms of educational work, and assistance to other families and to poor or handicapped children."[35] The problem for infertile believers is not in the suggestion that the longing for children of one's own can be tapped as an energy for service. It is in the dissonance between the high value placed on biological reproduction and the assumption that, being surrounded by and having taken in this interpretation of its significance, the infertile can simply reinterpret it.

Taking seriously the difficulty of this double message for the infertile calls for theological reconstruction in at least two ways. First, although describing reproduction as the "supreme," the "most gratuitous" gift of marriage[36] captures the sense in which our participation in reproduction is always an invitation into the mystery of God's creative action, the language of gift in this context implies a problematic passivity with respect to reproduction and a divine ratification of the fitness of the person or the marriage for reproduction. The important value of reproduction as cocreation can be better expressed in the language of "trust" or "stewardship" that underscores the intentional and reverent participation of the spouses in reproduction, without suggesting that children are distributed willy-nilly according to divine favor or whim. To say that our children are entrusted to us recognizes that, as human beings, formed *imago dei*, our children are not our possessions. To understand parenthood as a form of stewardship captures the sense of awe and responsibility that properly attends the event of bringing forth a distinct new life. At the same time, such language recognizes our intentional—rational as well as emotional—participation in the process of reproduction, offsetting the image of reproduction as a capricious event. Feminist criticisms of an overly mystical view of reproduction in the biblical traditions and of ongoing efforts to retrieve an emphasis on women's agency in reproduction are useful resources for the shift in language and perception I am suggesting here.

Also in need of reconstruction is the place of procreation in a theology of marriage. Contemporary theological treatments of the ends of marriage give equal importance to its unitive and procreative dimensions. But a continued emphasis on procreation as the "fullness" or "flowering" of marital intimacy, an emphasis that, as we have seen is readily internalized, tends to render the childless marriage "second class." Theologians such as Christine Gudorf have argued that the Christian tradition's failure to develop the unitive aspect of sexual love leaves a procreation-centered norm for sexual expression that has been both destructive of women's development within marriage and reproductively irresponsible.[37] As is clear from earlier chapters, it has been important here to retain a central place for the procreative dimension of sexual intimacy and for the theological significance of biological reproduction. Still, Gudorf and others are correct that Christian sexual ethics must shift from an inflated emphasis on the generation of life to an emphasis on the sustaining of life.[38] Elevating the significance of marriage as first and foremost for the mutual self-giving of the partners reflects more accurately the reality of married life and the place of procreation within it, as well as giving rise to a norm for reproduction that respects the conditions for healthy and responsible reproduction. To articulate a *genuine* theological significance to the achievement of a life-giving and generative but not necessarily procreative union between spouses also creates the context for helping infertile couples to celebrate their own relationship, which may be childless but need not be "sterile." I take as well a related caution: Christian sexual ethics is in need of a shift from an emphasis on the acquisition of children to an emphasis on the care of children. Where the procreative norm has encouraged a proprietary view of biological reproduction, it has not served children well and has interfered with a view of parenthood that would count the welcoming of children as highly as the "production" of children. Looking hard at what exactly we as Christians value in parenthood is necessary if we are to create a context in which we can commend adoption or other ways of relating to children as attractive paths to resolving the infertility crisis.

Still another obstacle to constructing a viable faith context for coping with infertility is our failure, at least in the Catholic Church, to develop fully the baptismal vocation of the laity. To privilege the family as the primary place of ministry for lay Catholics lends valuable support to the work of family life, but it has tended at the same time to eclipse the more fundamental call to ministry and service that all Christians share. It has the practical effect of making single Catholics and childless couples invisible, not only liturgically, but as a force for effective witness in the world. What is needed is a way of talking seriously about the call to faithfulness and action that follows directly from our baptism, which we all share, and which can be lived out in a variety of equally viable forms of life. What is needed, in other words, is a theology of lay vocation that treats single life or marriage without children as a unique and valuable context for ministry—not, as we tend to treat them now, simply as "holding patterns." It is only when we affirm the service of the laity in the church in its own right that we create a setting in which it makes sense to call the infertile beyond an intense desire for biological parenthood to generous service in the church and in the world.

At the end of her journey through infertility, as she decides that she will no longer pursue pregnancy, Alden recounts her turn to religion:

> *I hadn't been to church in years, but now I started visiting different churches. I wanted to be in a sacred place, and I wanted to hear someone speak of God's way, God's knowing, as opposed to human knowledge, or more specifically, my knowledge. In one church I visited, before the service people got up and lit slender tapers. I was moved by these people, touched by whatever grief or loss was in their hearts. I would have liked to go up and light a candle myself, but I was afraid to. I was afraid I'd break down.*[39]

This is precisely what is at stake for Christian ethics in calling for a greater awareness of potentially transformative liturgical moments and a re-thinking of the way we talk about the significance of procreation and parent-hood theologically: the offer of a "sacred place" for those trying to cope with infertility. To come forward as infertile, to face the reality that the ordinary pleasures and challenges of reproduction are not available to you, is an act of courage. As Rehner reminds us, it is the birth of freedom and the avenue to new possibilities for self-understanding. But coming forward, coming home to one's faith community, will only be the initiation of a spiritual quest, the opportunity for grasping the life that lies beyond infertility, if those communities take seriously infertility's toll. To recognize, with the infertile, what has been lost, not only of plans and expectations, but of the *self*, is the beginning of becoming a healing presence just as it is the beginning of healing.

NOTES

1 Arthur L. Greil, *Not Yet Pregnant: Infertile Couples in Contemporary America* (New Brunswick, N.J.: Rutgers University Press, 1991), 161ff.

2 I have borrowed this description from Paulette Bates Alden's *Crossing the Moon: A Journey through Infertility* (St. Paul, Minn.: Hungry Mind Press, 1996), 278.

3 Jan Rehner, *Infertility: Old Myths, New Meanings* (Toronto: Second Story Press, 1989), 112.

4 Eric Cassell, "The Nature of Suffering and the Goals of Medicine," *New England Journal of Medicine* 306, no. 11 (March 18, 1982): 642.

5 I am using the terms "infertility" and "barrenness" interchangeably here, although, of course, the terms do not have exactly the same meaning. In the biblical texts, for example, is not always clear whether "barrenness" refers simply to the state of not having borne children (i.e., "infertility") and/or to the state of not having born sons or descendents in the sense of followers in male lineage. However, both terms connote involuntary childlessness and it is in that sense that I am using them. All biblical references are taken from the Revised Standard Version (Cleveland, Ohio: The World Publishing Co., 1962).

6 Phyllis Trible, *God and the Rhetoric of Sexuality* (Philadelphia: Fortress Press, 1978), 34–35.

7 Ibid., 35.

8 Greil, *Not Yet Pregnant,* 167.

9 [http://www.hannah.org].

10 *Catechism of the Catholic Church*, no. 2366 (Washington, D.C.: United States Catholic Conference, 1994), 569.

11 John Paul II, *On the Dignity and Vocation of Women* (*Mulieris Dignitatem*) (Washington, D.C.: United States Catholic Conference, August 15, 1988), 111.

12 Although *Mulieris Dignitatem* describes consecrated virginity as "spiritual marriage."

13 *Catechism of the Catholic Church*, no. 2366, 569, 572.
14 Margaret A. Farley, "The Church and the Family: An Ethical Task," *Horizons*, 10, no. 1 (1983): 50–71.
15 *Catechism of the Catholic Church*, no. 2366, 569, 572.
16 Michael Kress, "Be Fruitful and Multiply," available at [http://www.salon.com/mwt/feature/2002/02/03/infertility].
17 See Greil, *Not Yet Pregnant,* 166ff.
18 Ibid., 171.
19 Ibid., 173.
20 Hannah's Prayer [http://www.hannah.org].
21 The founders of Hannah's Prayer, Richard and Jennifer Saake, make the important point that Mother's Day and Father's Day are civic rather than religious holidays and need not be celebrated at all. It seems to me that these holidays provide an opportunity to highlight a primary feature of life for most members of the congregation and a valued set of relationships within religious traditions. I would argue that they should not be celebrated liturgically only if they cannot be celebrated with sensitivity to the various forms of family life within the congregation as well as the vast differences of experiences of family present.
22 Julie Kelemen, *Dealing with Infertility: A Guide for Catholics* (Liguori, Mo.: Liguori Publications, 1997), 18.
23 Hugo Kugiya, "Having Faith: Service Devoted to Infertile Couples," *Seattle Times* (January 26, 1998), L1.
24 [http://www.hannah.org/church.htm].
25 Anita Goldman, "The Production of Eggs and the Will of God," in *Infertility: Women Speak Out about Their Experiences of Reproductive Medicine*, Renate D. Klein, ed. (London: Pandora Press, 1989), 72. Goldman is describing a treatment regimen where ovulation is the goal, the indicator of which would be an elevated body temperature. Whatever the procedures, however, ovulation and menstruation are the generally measured events, the common indicators of success or failure.
26 Rehner, *Infertility*, 20–21 (emphasis original). Rehner is quoting Carol Christ, *Diving Deep and Surfacing* (Boston: Beacon Press, 1980), 76.
27 Rehner, *Infertility,* 103.
28 Ibid., 104.
29 Ibid., 105.
30 Ibid., 115.
31 Alden, *Crossing the Moon*, 287.
32 Rehner, *Infertility,* 120.
33 Edmund D. Pellegrino and David C. Thomasma, *The Christian Virtues in Medical Practice* (Washington, D.C.: Georgetown University Press, 1996), 67–68.
34 Richard A. McCormick, "Theology and Bioethics," *Hastings Center Report* 19, no. 2, 5–10.

35 Congregation for the Doctrine of the Faith, "Instruction on Respect for Human Life in Its Origin and on the Dignity of Procreation: Replies to Certain Questions of the Day, *(Donum Vitae)*," (February 22, 1987), no. 8. As reprinted in *Gift of Life: Catholic Scholars Respond to the Vatican Document*, edited by Edmund D. Pellegrino, John Collins Harvey, and John P. Langan (Washington, D.C.: Georgetown University Press, 1990), 31.
36 Congregation for the Doctrine of the Faith, "Instruction," no. 8, 031.
37 Christine E. Gudorf, *Body, Sex and Pleasure: Reconstructing Christian Sexual Ethics* (Cleveland, Ohio: The Pilgrim Press, 1994).
38 Ibid., 129.
39 Alden, *Crossing the Moon*, 275.

CONCLUSION

Years ago, I told one of my professors that I was interested in writing on questions of justice in the allocation of health care. She replied that such questions made wonderful research topics in that so little had been well worked out. On the other hand, she went on to say, they made terrible research topics, as it was nearly impossible to work them out to anyone's satisfaction, let alone everyone's satisfaction.

Our look at access to assisted reproduction bears out the truth of her observation. Whether or not infertile couples have a right to assisted reproduction in a just health care system is a rich and multilayered question, touching on the meaning of health and disease, the social function of medicine, the place of reproduction in accounts of human flourishing, and the limits of social commitments to personal well-being. It is also an inescapably complex question, to which any answer will be provisional, partial, and in the end, disappointing.

The way we resolve problems—whether social or personal—has a great deal to do with the way we have defined them. If we think that we have unlimited resources at our disposal, our range of alternatives also appears unlimited. If we see our problem or crisis as unique, individual, and isolated, we are free to consider alternatives as though our choices mattered for no one but ourselves. Although the problem of involuntary childlessness is often construed in exactly this way, we have seen that neither assumption can hold. The resources with which to meet the basic needs of people in this country and in the world are not unlimited, and the choices of individuals concerning reproduction have serious social consequences.

By placing the issue of assisted reproduction within the context of the common good, where justice is understood in terms of guaranteeing a basic level of participation, we have been able to ask what a choice to pursue sophisticated and expensive infertility treatment means in light of obligations to guarantee all persons basic access to the conditions for a meaningful life within the community. In this framework, where all human rights are relative and reciprocal, the freedom to pursue medically assisted reproduction is assessed along with other claims on the community, such as claims to basic health care, dignified work, economic initiative, and adequate food and housing. Concerned with the conditions that marginalize persons in various ways, for example, within economic and political systems, the health care system, and within social communities of meaning and identity, we have attempted to see infertility in its complex relationship to other constitutive features of human well-being. As a dimension of human flourishing, the opportunity to conceive or bear a child of one's own can be called basic without being necessary, central without being essential.

Viewing infertility as a matter of human well-being, of health considered as part of a capacity for agency, allows us to ask of reproductive technologies the kinds of questions asked of other health care goods, such as the ratio of benefit to burden, the place of this technology in the table of health care priorities, the importance of a medical over a nonmedical solution for a certain kind of problem, and whether it is caring or curing that matters in a particular case.

However, as we have seen, there are trade-offs in adopting this approach. To give "reproductive impairment" a claim to medical energies and resources, however relative to other claims, emphasizes the ability to impregnate, to bear and bring forth a child, to reproduce biologically. We cannot help but take up an ideal that has become increasingly problematic, both for the pride of place it gives to the generation of children verses the care of children, and its role in encouraging a history of women's reproductive servitude. To respond to the articulated experience of infertile individuals, to act on what they express about the importance of biological reproduction in their lives, seems inevitably to involve promoting values we have good reason to question. At the very least we seem to be playing into the social construction of their need.

Moreover, it appears impossible to argue for the value of a medical solution to infertility without further medicalizing reproduction. It is an ironic feature of assisted reproduction that it makes reproductive self-determination, reproductive agency, possible only by handing oneself over to the experts. Feminists have long worried about the risks to women of such a submersion of the self in the technical process of assisted reproduction. To give up control this way, they have warned, leaves women, individually and collectively, particularly vulnerable to exploitation in the service of others' interests. But it is not only control that is at risk in the medicalization of infertility. It is also the obligations of care. Just as in other types of medicine, the personal is easily lost in the quest for cure, or in this case, for a child.

But it could be argued that the challenge to analyze assisted reproduction has been issued to the entire health care system today. It is not just with regard to infertility that an effort must be made to attend to, and distinguish between, the particular suffering of persons and the social construction of their experience. Not only involuntary childlessness, but illness, disability, and death in general are lived within certain social meanings that frame both the way needs are expressed by patients and the responses offered. It is not just those who cannot bear children who suffer losses defined by social expectations; so, too, do cancer patients who can no longer work, athletes who can no longer perform, and once-independent adults who can no longer care for their own needs. And it is not just the infertile whose anguish is vulnerable to exploitation; collective fears about death and loss of control are continually tapped to feed and sustain the immense health care industry in the United States.

Therefore, whether in reproductive medicine or health care in general, the challenge to see things from "both places at once," to respond to particular patients *within* their environment, is inescapable for those whose ultimate concern is equitable care. Health care goals and priorities are established in the complex relationship between what is demanded, what is possible, what is offered, and what is finally affordable. In light of the ambiguous character of reproductive technologies and pressing obligations of equity, we have called here for a sort of humility with respect to what ought to be demanded as well as what ought to be promised. But for such a response to be just, we have argued that it must be possible for individuals, especially for women, to retain or reconstruct the self that is threatened by involuntary childlessness. Thus a healing of the conditions of possibility for health care choices is inseparable from the healing of persons. It is this kind of "environmental" reform, open and honest attention to the reasons why health and health care is important to societies as well as to individuals, that will ultimately be necessary across the board if persons in the United States are going to be well cared for, if technology is to be developed and employed responsibly, and if reasonable limits are to be set.

Exactly how to make the health care system accountable to the common good is matter of great debate. What package of services should be considered a "decent minimum," how much inequality in receipt of services can be tolerated within a commitment to provide universal access, and whether the option to buy out of a basic plan inevitably preserves freedom of choice at the price of equality are questions that even readers of the same tradition, for example, Roman Catholic social teaching, can answer quite differently. How to bring the fertility industry under the umbrella of accountability is also a matter of debate. Although we have not addressed the question of regulation in our discussion, it is a critical question that will ultimately have to be faced in this country. The strong weight of American traditions of procreative liberty and the current independence of fertility clinics will make it extremely difficult to attempt to place external constraints on the practices of assisted reproduction.

And yet it is obvious that we cannot talk about orienting assisted reproductive technologies toward the common good without facing its current "Wild West" character. We might imagine various possibilities for bringing moderating influences to bear, from following the lead of other countries in adopting federal guidelines for assisted reproduction, to using reimbursement strategies to encourage compliance with practice standards. Whatever mechanisms we adopt, however, it will be necessary to do more than give lip service to the interests of children. The rights of potential offspring and the rights of would-be parents are not in necessary opposition, but neither are they simply collapsible one into the other as our current practices suggest.

We have set the questions of access to assisted reproduction within a larger vision for reforming the health care system. In doing so, we run the risk of offering a doubly unsatisfying answer to the questions of justice with which we began. The adoption of an ethical framework in which the values of self-determination and equality are equally compelling, and where the needs and interests of particular persons are juxtaposed to the goals of creating conditions for a "good human life in communion" requires placing a great deal of trust in the power of human solidarity. Ultimately, we recognize that the crucial locus for accountability is in the demands we bring to the system and the choices we make with respect to the resources available to us. The hope for a health care system that is "temperate, affordable, sustainable, and equitable" lies in the capacity to recognize the interconnection of needs and the consequences of choices for the whole. As such, we are presupposing not only that it is possible to call social systems and patterns of distribution to accountability in light of shared human needs, but also that individuals are capable of making community-oriented and community-responsive choices, for example, about the use of health care goods—and of accepting limitations for the sake of the common good. In this sense, hope may rest on a fragile foundation indeed.

It is both the fragility of this hope and the inescapable ambiguity of assisted reproductive technologies that explain why this book ended where it did, with a look at resources in the Christian tradition for healing and transcendence in the face of infertility. Ultimately, the possibilities for a just and responsible use of reproductive technologies lie in the creation of a social climate where personal worth is not defined by being able to produce offspring and where a moral and healthy choice can be made to relinquish the privileges of economic power in favor of a less costly alternative, a less immediately desirable option. There is a vision of a larger family of which we are all part in the Christian tradition, a family of humankind that can take us beyond an unhealthy focus on the biological family; there is a vision of an eternal self, a self that is fulfilled not in this world but in God, that can take us past the limits of mortal illness and impairment.

But through the glimpses we have given of the experience of infertility, it should be possible to see that no one is free to make a hard choice, or even a responsible one, so long as the price of infertility is so high. Persons who feel abnormal, asexual, and incomplete, and who believe they have been cheated out of an opportunity that is nonetheless required of them, will find it difficult to be great hearted. In the social construction of the infertility crisis are the clues to the social healing of infertility: a reinterpretation of the connections between sexuality and reproduction, a refashioning of the meanings of generativity and fruitfulness, a reassessment of the place of genetic relation in our understandings of parenthood, and a deepening of women's and men's self-understanding beyond maternity and paternity. Still, the courage to open one's heart to a child who needs you more than you need him, to take loss and disappointment and make of them an opportunity for solidarity, and, most important, to learn and share the lesson infertility teaches about finitude and humility, is a spiritual capacity, born in the reassurance that one's loss is honored even while life beyond loss is being called forth.

Too often, our response to the ambiguities of infertility and assisted reproduction is to try to convince those affected that their longing is not real or that it can be easily turned into another form. Not only will that approach fail, it does violence to the hunger that, however questionable the forces that shape it, is "not a belief, but a certainty."

Index